Praise for
Shattering

Marcie Jones is an exceptional writer. The story is beautifully told. She really knows how to involve the reader.

—Dr. Ken West
Professor Emeritus of Counseling and Human Development,
University of Lynchburg

Shattering is wonderful. It is well written and will be a comfort for families going through similar trials.

—Gretchen Fincke, LCSW, CST
Psychotherapist

I am so moved by *Shattering*. It's a powerful memoir of a mother's undying love, faith, family, challenges, and the profound human spirit. I was compelled from page to page, not wanting to take breaks. This book is powerful and relevant to many families who have walked similar troubling paths. It provides inspiration and dedication to faith and connection.

—Joan Marineau, CAP
Licensed Mental Health Counselor

What an amazing journey outlined in an emotional outpouring of love, faith, and support. I was deeply moved by the intense love of family and friends. Hunter is lucky to have Marcie as his mom and to have a family dedicated to supporting him.

I believe all things happen for a reason, although we cannot see it at the time. Marcie's willingness to share her story—just like her willingness in the depths of pain to sit with, hold hands with, listen to, and pray with Simone in the hospital family room—will touch someone and give them the strength and hope to make it through their challenges. I love Marcie's connections to Bible verses and to words of encouragement.

—Dr. Martha J. Eagle
Division Superintendent of Schools
Nelson County Public Schools, Virginia

Shattering is a gripping, compelling, and intimate narrative about the ultimate parenting challenge of living with the outcomes of a child's mental health issues. This is a must-read for anyone experiencing unsettling and seemingly insurmountable circumstances. Marcie Jones's compassionate memoir illustrates how family, faith, and perseverance transform tragedy into wins through small gains one day at a time.

—Ann M. Martin
Retired School Library Administrator
Past President, the American Association of School Librarians

Shattering

Shattering

Marcie S. Jones

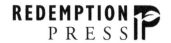
REDEMPTION PRESS

Published by Redemption Press, PO Box 427, Enumclaw, WA 98022
Toll Free (844) 2REDEEM (273-3336)

Redemption Press is honored to present this title in partnership with the author. The views expressed or implied in this work are those of the author. Redemption Press provides our imprint seal representing design excellence, creative content and high quality production.

This book is a memoir. It reflects the author's present recollections of experiences over time. Some events have been compressed, and some dialogue has been recreated. The names *Simone* and *Marie* were used to protect those individuals' identities. All other names in this book are real and are used with permission.

Author photo: Karen Smith

ISBN 13: 978-1-68314-802-9
ePub ISBN: 978-1-68314-803-6
Kindle ISBN: 978-1-68314-804-3
Library of Congress Catalog Card Number: 2019934496

A story from my heart for those in my heart . . .

Table of Contents

Prologue...11

Chapter 1 13

Chapter 2 17

Chapter 3 33

Chapter 4 51

Chapter 5 53

Chapter 6 57

Chapter 7 59

Chapter 8 61

Chapter 9 63

Chapter 10 69

Chapter 11 73

Chapter 12 77

Chapter 13 81

Chapter 14 85

Chapter 15 89

Chapter 16 93

Chapter 17 97

Chapter 18 101

Chapter 19 105

Chapter 21 109

Chapter 22 117

Chapter 23 121

Chapter 24 123

Chapter 25 129

Chapter 26 133

Chapter 27 137

Chapter 28 141

Chapter 29 145

Chapter 30 149

Chapter 31 155

Epilogue 157

Prologue

I'm shattering.
Day by day.
Breath by breath.
Heartbeat by heartbeat.
Just like the windshield.

The windshield on which my son threw himself in an effort to end his anguish and his life.

I still see the patterns that his head left on the glass. I still see him running. I see him picking his long, lean body off the lush summer grass and slamming his head into the tinted safety glass only to bounce off like an old-fashioned rubber ball.

That day, I stood alone, shocked, with one thought in my mind: *What should I do?*

I knew with certainty that whatever happened next would be worse.

It was.

Chapter 1

The back door snapped shut behind me with a click as I hurried out of the crisp fall air to embrace the warmth of our kitchen.

"Boo, I'm home," I called to my husband.

The ringing phone drowned out his response.

The words on Caller ID read *Hawaii.*

A niggle of anxiety wrapped around my heart as I picked up the phone. Our middle son lived on the Big Island, but he never called midweek.

I listened intently as a stranger's voice said, "Hi, Marcie, this is Charlie. Your son Hunter works for me."

Charlie owned Wailapa Farms, the organic coffee plantation where Hunter worked. He was teaching Hunter valuable lessons in how to raise the best Kona coffee on the island. Hunter always spoke highly of Charlie. He clearly admired him as a professional and a friend.

My mind tried to focus on Charlie's words about erratic behavior, a downward spiral, and rants about bees. They made no sense.

By the time Charlie got to "rushed to Kona Community Hospital," my husband was standing beside me, looking perplexed and concerned. After hanging up, I repeated as much of the phone conversation as I could recall, then dialed the number Charlie had just given me.

That was when I learned something that tore at my heart even more than the reality that Hunter had been admitted to the hospital.

The nurse would not provide more information about his condition. HIPAA laws prevented it.

"Please, we are thousands of miles away. Can't you tell me anything?" I begged.

"I can't without his permission," the nurse replied. She sounded empathetic. "I can tell you he is here and that we will try to get him to sign the HIPAA form so we can release information to you."

That night was one of the longest in my life.

It was difficult enough to learn that Hunter was having a mental health crisis, but now I had to tell his brother and sister, Michael and Bridget. Our children were adults, yet their pain cut into my soul as I shared the news and tried to soothe them long distance.

As my husband and I prepared for bed, we prayed fervently for Hunter. We asked God to comfort Michael and Bridget and give us guidance for how to help our son. The night brought little sleep, but Boo and I managed to drag ourselves out of bed and to work. That day felt even longer than the night before. As an administrator at a small Christian school, I had office duties and teaching responsibilities. How would I keep my middle and high school students on track with their grammar and literature classes without falling apart? I needed to tell my parents about Hunter and keep Michael and Bridget updated. But most importantly, I had to talk to Hunter. St. Paul's advice in 1 Thessalonians to "pray without ceasing" (ASV) became the glue that held me together as I put one foot in front of the other and kept going.

The nurse I'd talked to the night before finally called.

"Mrs. Jones, Hunter has signed the HIPAA papers." The knot in my heart loosened a tiny bit, and I let out a breath I didn't realize I'd been holding. Finally, I could get some answers. Because of his precarious mental condition, Hunter couldn't talk to me yet, but knowing about his condition provided a degree of solace. *Thank you, Lord*, I prayed.

Holding back tears, I rapidly scribbled notes as the nurse described the state in which Hunter had been brought to the emergency room. He'd arrived covered in bee stings, severely dehydrated, malnourished, and hallucinating. He thought he had implants in his teeth and that they were picking up transmissions. Blood tests revealed marijuana in his system. The nurse explained that the cannabis on the island was particularly potent and might have been laced with a hallucinogenic.

She said Hunter's psychotic break was so severe that it required a sedative injected into his leg and eleven hospital staff to remove him from the truck he arrived in. That image alone shook me to my core. Growing up, Hunter had rarely been aggressive. He had decked a fellow kindergartener on the playground, but only because the boy pushed Hunter's friend off the swing. Other than that, he'd been an easygoing kid.

After hanging up with the nurses, I called Charlie. I still needed to fit the pieces of this puzzle together.

"Hi, Charlie. It's Marcie. I just talked to one of the nurses at the hospital." The words rushed out of my mouth. "How could this happen? Hunter was fine the last time I talked to him. I don't understand."

Charlie, a doctor by profession, recalled the week before Hunter's break.

"Hunter was one hundred percent normal until Sunday afternoon, when I noticed he seemed a little off. By Monday he was confused and anxious. He made inappropriate comments to some mainland visitors, which was out of character for him. By Wednesday he got even worse, and I wondered if he was stressed beyond what he could handle."

As I tried to comprehend all this happening to my son, Charlie continued, "I finally asked him how he was feeling. He told me that something wasn't quite right, but he didn't know what, so I left it alone thinking things would return to normal. They didn't."

By Thursday Hunter's world came crashing down. Now he lay in a hospital and I sat at home helplessly waiting to talk to him.

Chapter 2

It took several days for Hunter's mental state to tilt toward stable. Saturday dawned and the phone rang.

"Hi, Mom."

I knew that voice, despite its hesitancy and confusion.

"Hi, Hunter. It's so good to hear you. How are you feeling?"

I cringed at my words. How did I expect him to be after what happened? But it was a question only Hunter could answer.

"I'm not good, Mom. I'm in a hospital here in Kona. I don't remember everything that happened, but I am doing what they tell me. I was flying with the bees and pollinating flowers. I had to do it. The voices were telling me to."

Hunter continued in a thready, frightened tone. "They are still talking to me. They are telling me that I can only walk on the black squares in the hospital, so I am jumping from square to square."

I felt my legs slowly give out beneath me as I processed what Hunter was telling me. I gracelessly slid into the nearest kitchen chair. *Breathe in . . . breathe out*, I told myself. *Lord, give me words.*

The Lord gave Hunter words instead. "The food is good here. And I like the nurses."

His words made the remainder of our conversation easier to handle.

It was those nurses who first learned that Hunter had been hearing voices since college. He identified the voices as the Holy Spirit and followed the directives, whether they were good or harmful.

How had we missed this? How had *I* missed it? When Hunter was in college, my husband and I had visited and talked to him on a regular basis. His college years had started out fairly well—he served as a resident advisor during his sophomore year. After that, he took a job caring for a retired university instructor who had Alzheimer's disease. During the first few months of this job, Hunter went to the professor's house and walked with him or just sat with him. He talked with the professor's wife and developed a great respect for her. As time passed and the disease ravaged the professor, Hunter moved into the couple's basement apartment so he could be more readily available. He grew to love and admire them both. The professor's death hit Hunter hard. He had helped the elderly man for so long that he thought of him as another grandfather and mourned him as one. Eventually, Hunter decided he couldn't finish college and asked to rent his grandma's old house up the road from us so he could start a computer business.

Like college, the business never quite worked out. After a few months, he'd moved to Hawaii.

Were these the red flags I couldn't see?

Beating myself up now while Hunter suffered so many miles away would not help him or me. At this point, the doctors couldn't even tell us if Hunter's psychotic break was caused by cannabis or a mental illness. They labeled it as an adjustment disorder with mood and conduct and put him on several different medicines. I felt like I was drowning in foreign terms. After learning that an adjustment disorder was a person's inability to adapt to any number of stressors and could cause depression, anxiety, and behavioral problems, I immediately researched the names of the drugs Hunter was taking: Geodon, Zyprexa, Topamax. These were the first of many high-powered meds that I became familiar with. I understood their value, but I also became aware of their debilitating side effects.

Each day presented us with a new challenge. The most immediate one became finding a way to get Hunter home to Virginia.

His brother had already thought about this. He called to tell me, "Mom, I'll go to Hawaii to get Hunter. I can talk to his doctors and find out more about his situation. Then we can figure out a way to get him home." Michael booked a flight from his home in

Portland, Oregon, took several days off from work, and headed to Kona.

One of Hunter's friends allowed Michael to stay with him. Michael spent sleepless nights on that friend's living room floor and days watching his anxiety-filled brother's distress. Each day was different as Hunter's behavior vacillated between rational and erratic. Michael kept me updated through phone calls and email.

"We had a great visit today, Mom. We laughed a lot about things we did as kids and talked about home."

Then on another day he reported, "Today wasn't a good one for Hunter. He was bouncing around again, going from one linoleum square to another and mumbling about a voice telling him what to do. It was hard to see him that way."

And then the call we had been waiting and praying for came.

"The doctor will let Hunter leave with me."

We arranged side-by-side seats for Michael and Hunter on the flight to Portland and a nonstop flight from Portland to Washington, DC. Armed with a week's worth of medication, they landed in Oregon. The first thing they did was get Hunter a haircut and some new clothes. The hope was that these would give him some added confidence as he flew across country by himself.

Bridget and her husband, Marcus, picked him up in DC and drove him to Charlottesville, where Boo and I met them at a restaurant.

For over a week, my prayer had been for the Lord to be with Hunter and bring him healing. When I saw him in Charlottesville, I added another prayer: *Dear God, please help us to help Hunter.*

Haunted was the thought that ran through my mind as I hugged my son for the first time in months. His closely cropped red hair framed his gaunt face. His eyes were filled with fear. He looked thinner than he had ever been, even as a high school student trying to make weight for wrestling. He smiled at me across the restaurant table, and my heart caught in my throat. Could I make it through the meal without crying?

Could I make it through the following weeks?

We had Hunter with us, but he wasn't the same young man who'd left home a couple of years earlier. He wanted to return to Hawaii and talked about it constantly. We understood his desire, but we also believed he would recuperate faster by staying in Virginia, close to family. This became a point of contention as the days progressed.

"Hawaii is my home. Thank you for your help, but I want to go home."

"I know you miss Hawaii, Hunter, but you don't have anyone to help you there. You have to get better. You need to be with us."

"But this isn't my home anymore. I want to go to Hawaii."

Adjusting to his medications only made things harder. Hunter's meds were supposed to help his psychosis, but they also affected his thinking, his walking, and his speech. I understood his frustration. What twenty-seven-year-old wanted his head to feel like it was filled with cotton and to shuffle his feet like an old man? Not only did he not like the side effects, but he also couldn't afford them without insurance, which he didn't have.

After only six days at home, Hunter landed in another behavioral treatment center. His doctor in Hawaii had told me that it could take a few weeks for the medicine to be fully effective, and that proved to be true. We had driven to Lynchburg to meet with a mental health professional to see what services were available to Hunter and at what cost. The closer we drove to the therapist's office, the more nervous and agitated Hunter became. He wanted to return to Hawaii. Despite having a major psychotic break there, he felt compelled to return. We walked into the building, signed in, and waited to be seen. Suddenly, Hunter got up and walked out the door.

Trying to tamp down my panic, I called out to him. "Hunter, where are you going?"

"I have to go to Hawaii," he replied in a monotone. "It's my home."

Oh, my gosh, I thought. *He's having another break right in front of my eyes.*

Within a short time, my husband had joined me, and we both talked with the therapist. We needed to find Hunter. Given his statement about returning to Hawaii, we believed he might try to walk to the airport, but we had no idea what route he would use. The counselor suggested that the best thing for Hunter's safety was to involve law enforcement in searching for him. It was both abhorrent and heartbreaking to even think this was necessary, but the fact was that Hunter was on heavy antipsychotic meds and had only been out of mental health unit a little over a week. I was terrified for his safety.

Shortly after the police began their search, Hunter was picked up and taken to a local hospital. Boo and I met him there and came face to face with his anger. He could not understand that we had asked the police to find him for his own safety. He felt betrayed and believed we wanted to keep him a prisoner.

Oh, Lord, please help us to help our son, I prayed as we listened to a doctor tell us that Hunter would be placed in a behavioral unit in a hospital in another city.

This facility might have been closer to us in proximity than the one in Hawaii, but it was still not what I'd envisioned for Hunter. I had naively believed that the high-powered meds would bring stability and healing.

So began the first in a series of email updates to Boo, Michael, and Bridget.

Good morning to all of you, I just spoke with the charge nurse on Hunter's floor. He is up and in "group" just now. He is confused and has to have things explained to him again before he processes them. Even though he signed himself in, he doesn't want to be there.

We don't want to force ourselves on him and cause more agitation, so we're trying to let him make the first move. The nurse said Hunter would definitely be there for five days and she believes he will be in a behavioral unit for a week or more. The facility could change due to his lack of insurance. The insurance folks at the hospital could have him moved to a state facility after the five days. I pray they keep him here because I don't think a change of locale is good for him. I believe it would be more beneficial if he continued with the same psychiatrist until a somewhat definitive diagnosis is determined.

As to what they are looking at: the charge nurse indicated bipolar and schizophrenia. The doctor has noted both of them as possibilities. It will take a while to be certain. In the meantime, keep praying that God will be with the doctor as he makes his observations and diagnosis and that Hunter can begin to have mental clarity.

Bridget is driving in today. I will ride with her to visit Hunter. Boo and I agree that I should wait in the waiting area and have Bridget ask if Hunter wants to see me. If he does, I'll go in. Otherwise I'll just wait outside for the duration.

I plan to take clothes again today to see if Hunter wants them. As much clothes washing as he did during his few days here, I would think he would like a change. Of course, he was thinking more clearly a few days ago.

We'll let you know how the day goes.

Thank you for your help and prayers.

Love,

Mama

When Bridget arrived home later that morning, we ate an early lunch and started the hour and a half drive to LewisGale Hospital in Salem.

After the previous day's visit, I wasn't certain what to expect. I tried to mentally prepare myself for the possibility that Hunter wouldn't want to see me. But as soon as we entered the ward and greeted him, his green eyes lit up and he wrapped his arms around me. I held in grateful tears as my heart swelled.

Bridget and Hunter visited in his room while I stayed at the nurses' station and waited for them to inspect the items I'd brought. The hospital had numerous rules about what patients could have. I tried hard to adhere to them. Hunter's list of requests included homemade cookies, venison, cornbread, nuts, and granola, as well as fresh clothing, his own toothbrush and toothpaste, and some books and pictures. Luckily, everything I brought met the hospital criteria, so I put them back in the tote and walked to Hunter's room.

Despite his warm greeting when we first arrived, the minute I entered his room he made it clear he wanted to go home. He could not understand why he needed to be in the hospital.

"The place is full of crazies, and I'm not one of them. I'm taking my meds. Why won't they let me go?"

Bridget replied before I could formulate my thoughts. "Hunter, I don't know why they won't release you, but we're doing what we think is best. We love you and only want what is best for you,"

"But my home is in Hawaii, and I want to go back there," he insisted.

Once again my spirits plummeted. While I had always believed that our adult children needed to find happiness wherever they chose to live, I fervently wished he had never gone to Hawaii.

In an email to her dad and Michael, Bridget described the rest of our visit.

We found out from the nurses as we were leaving that it's OK to tell Hunter what the docs are looking into and we can bring him material regarding the disorders for him to read through. I don't know what the doctor has told him. From what I get from Hunter, the doc said he needs to stop being so eccentric. He told me that his home is in Hawaii and he wanted to go back there. I asked him if he missed us and he said "No." (I know this was the illness talking, because he called me from HI homesick a few times. I know he missed us!) I asked him where he'd live in HI and he said he had a tarp. Basically, he's still set on going back . . . We had also spoken about my flowers (which were budding, amazingly because we'd already had a frost!). I cut those flowers and brought them to Hunter today and he didn't recall our conversation or ever seeing the flowers at my house. I've really noticed his memory has been affected—long and short term.

I am going back down tomorrow before I go back to my house and am hoping for a much more "Hawaii-free Hunter." He is truly obsessed with getting back. Mom's going to piggy back with me since we know that she'll be received. Hopefully, he'll be able to recognize some of the symptoms for the disorders we're printing off and it will help him to understand. He told us both that he loves us and was receptive to the hugs and wanted to know if I'd come back tomorrow. The doc did tell Hunter that there was a 99% chance he would not be able to get out today. Hunter's response to us about that is that there's a 1% chance he WILL be released (I have to admit, I love positive thinking).

All in all, I really wished the visit had gone better, but it was so good to get his hugs and hear him say he loves us. To me, that's a small step better than yesterday, so hopefully he'll keep getting better and better.

Love,

Bridget

These days were as difficult for all of us as when Hunter was hospitalized in Hawaii. He just wasn't our Hunter. We prayed, talked, and held in tears, but we could not take away his pain and confusion.

We continued to email Charlie with updates. His insight as a physician helped as we navigated a mental health system fraught with flaws that included lengthy delays in patients seeing psychiatrists and lack of information on how to secure help.

The ringing of the phone startled me as I set the table for dinner one evening, thinking about Hunter. The plan was to eat an early meal, then drive to Salem to visit with him. We were hoping to get an update from the doctor.

Instead, it was Hunter calling. "Mom, can I stay with you and Daddy tonight if they let me out?"

I carefully responded, "I don't think they are going to discharge you today, Hunter. But you can stay with us whenever you get out. You can stay for more than one night."

"Okay, but it will only be short term. I am an adult and can make my own decisions." His tone challenged me to disagree.

"You're right. You can." I couldn't dispute his statement about being an adult. He needed all the confidence he could muster. But in his current mental state, trusting him with decision-making was going to be a challenge.

"I love you, Mom."

"I love you too, Hunter."

As we hung up, random thoughts raced through my mind. With each one, I sent specific prayers to the heavens. It must have been so hard for Hunter to ask if he could stay with us. If he felt uncertain that he would have a place to stay, his anxiety ran deep. *Lord, how could he even think that he would not be welcome at home?*

I discovered the answer to that question when I spoke to one of the nurses on Hunter's floor. She commented that we visited more than relatives of other patients. When I expressed my surprise, she explained that many patients were discharged from behavioral health units with nowhere to go. She told me, "As the patients get older and have more mental health issues, their families get tired of trying to help. They give up and close their doors to their loved ones."

Please God, I prayed, *give us the strength to always help our son when he needs us, no matter what the circumstances.*

As Hunter's days in the hospital continued, a diagnosis eluded the doctors. They needed more time to observe him and see how the meds affected him, but at the same time, the health care system didn't allow uninsured patients to spend weeks in a hospital. Patients like Hunter filed for financial help. In most cases the hospital absorbed the cost, which provided much-needed help for those who could not afford it otherwise. I don't know what we would have done if Hunter had been released during these psychotic episodes.

During a family meeting before Hunter's release, his doctors shared their possible diagnosis: schizoaffective disorder with OCD and generalized anxiety. They added Trazodone and Propranolol to the drug regimen that already included Geodon, Zyprexa, and Topamax. We were concerned about how to get ongoing mental health services for Hunter. When I called to schedule an appointment for him, the first available was more than two months out. The idea of him waiting that long terrified me.

Boo and I made a decision that we hoped would help Hunter more than we could. Rather than take him home with us, we would take him to stay with one of my brothers in Richmond. John and his wife, Carol, had started a peer-to-peer recovery program called the McShin Foundation. John, along with another brother, Peter, helped those with drug addictions and those with dual diagnoses, such as addiction with bipolar. The doctors had identified marijuana as a possible reason for Hunter's first psychotic episode in Hawaii, and we felt that John could help him. Hunter and John had always gotten along, so Hunter agreed to this solution.

The trip to Richmond flip-flopped between being relaxed and tense. We bounced from discussing everyday topics and how family members were doing to disagreeing about Hunter's need to stay on meds.

"I don't like the way they make me feel."

"I know," I told him, "and I am sorry, but you can't go off them now. We have to see if they'll help you get better." I empathized with Hunter, but I had to help him understand the importance of the drugs to his recovery.

I continued with my pep talk. "Uncle John and Aunt Carol have made an appointment for you to see one of the best psychiatrists in

Richmond. You can talk with him about the meds. Aunt Carol said you will really like him. His name is Dr. Master."

"What will I do in Richmond?" Hunter asked.

"Uncle John will take you with him to McShin," I explained. "You can help him with computer-related things. He'll make sure you go to NA meetings so you can start on the road to recovery."

Silence.

"Mom," he finally said. "Why didn't you tell me that I was born with a tail and had to have an operation to remove it?"

Boo shot a startled glance in my direction. He had been quiet for most of the trip. That was his way of coping, and it made it easier for him to focus on the crowded interstate.

I couldn't speak. Dread filled me. Where did he get such a thing? Was he having another episode? Did he really believe the story about having a tail?

"Hunter, you were not born with a tail. What makes you say that?"

"Michael told me when we were little. And I have an indentation at the base of my spine where it was removed."

Though stunned by Hunter's unexpected comment, the scientific term emerged from the recesses of my memory. "Hunter, that is a pilonidal dimple. You were born with it. It's an inherited trait." Hunter had always been our logical child, so I expected him to accept it without hesitation.

"No," he emphatically replied. "It's where you had my tail cut off."

I couldn't continue this conversation. Hunter truly believed the story, and I had no words to convince him otherwise.

Tamping down my rising anxiety, I prayed during much of the trek to Richmond. How would Hunter do at John's?

It didn't take long to find out.

Two days later, we received another phone call.

"Marcie, it's Peter." My brother's tone told me the news was not good.

Peter had the unenviable task of breaking the news of Hunter's latest psychotic episode. His voice cracked as he recalled the events of the evening. The McShin Foundation had hosted a pre-Thanksgiving meal for its residents, and Hunter was helping out with it. At some point, he had began jumping around in the building. He then ran outside and hid in the bushes, yelling that "they" were coming to get him. John and Peter tried to calm him, but the psychosis had a firm grip on Hunter, which made it impossible for him to process anything other than what the voices in his head were telling him. Once again, the police had to be called. My brothers went with Hunter to the hospital and stayed with him until 1:30 in the morning, waiting for him to stabilize.

Hunter finally looked at Peter and asked a question that tore at both my brothers: "There's something wrong with me then?"

Peter nodded and explained that river water can run straight or in swirls and eddies, and that at this point Hunter's thinking was like the swirls and eddies. Hunter seemed to grasp this analogy and nodded in acknowledgment.

How could Hunter continue to endure these psychotic episodes? They were destroying him and us. I worried for his mental and physical health. And I dreaded the ring of the phone because it no longer guaranteed a friendly voice wanting a casual conversation. It could be the voice of a stranger telling me that our cherished son was once again in the throes of a mental breakdown.

Charlie stayed in close communication with us after Hunter arrived in Virginia, so I sent him an email update after Peter's phone call.

Dear Charlie,

Hunter is currently in the Behavioral Unit at St. Mary's Hospital under sedation. We were planning to go to Richmond tomorrow for Thanksgiving and will still keep to this plan. We will visit Hunter and try to gain more information. I have no idea if he can or will sign a HIPAA allowing us to stay informed.

John is quite adept at dealing with this kind of trauma, and I pray he will continue to be able to help us. At this point, Dr. Master stated that he felt we were looking at one of three things: marijuana induced psychosis, bipolar, or schizophrenia. Hunter was supposed to visit another specialist on Friday to rule out schizophrenia. We hope the hospital will be able to follow up with this.

I suppose we are probably looking at a longer-term commitment. I'm not sure what the law says or what the medical regulations are, but based on what has happened over the past few days, I suspect a hearing will be held and that Hunter will be in a mental facility for a period of time that will allow him to be treated. As I said, I just don't know.

We will continue to keep you updated.

Marcie

Boo and I spent a subdued Thanksgiving with my family in Richmond, then went to visit Hunter at the hospital. When I finally wrapped my arms around my son, I wished my hug could make his nightmare disappear. He was in pain. We were in pain. Whatever was causing these psychotic episodes, the result was the same: chaos, anxiety, and confusion.

Boo stopped to talk with Hunter's nurses about his progress, and I joined Hunter in the visiting area.

"Mom," Hunter said after we sat down. "I am not hearing voices."

"That's good, Hunter," I assured him.

"No, you don't understand. I am not hearing voices!"

I finally figured out what he meant and was astounded at the revelation. Until that moment, I had not fully comprehended the fact that, for over five years, Hunter had been hearing voices that dictated what he said, did, and thought. Knowing he no longer heard them, I wanted to jump up and dance around the visiting room. I wanted to shout, "Thank you, Lord!" Hunter finally had peace in his mind for the first time since his early twenties. The change in meds had worked. Instead, I listened as Hunter described what it had been like for him, especially over the past month. His memory, both short term and long term, had been impaired, but he no longer felt like a voice was controlling his thoughts and actions.

Later, I wrote to my kids:

Dear Michael and Bridget,

I spoke with Hunter's psychiatrist over the phone earlier this evening and asked about his diagnosis/prognosis. I was surprised when the psychiatrist told me that he could not give us one. He said that patients must be observed for six months to two years to give a definitive diagnosis. Hunter could have schizophrenia, bipolar, or schizoaffective disorder, all of which terrify me. The doctor also said that he considers the past three-plus weeks one psychotic break and describes it as "psychosis not otherwise specified," a term used in Hawaii also.

"Hunter has responded extremely quickly and positively to the meds and 'schizos' do not respond this quickly," the doctor added. "Last week I would have bet $1,000 that Hunter had schizophrenia, but this week I just don't know. Time will tell the story."

Until today, I didn't know that a person could have a predisposition to schizophrenia. It seems that Hunter might and that the Hawaiian marijuana triggered the first break. Later in our conversation, I asked if Hunter had told him that he had been hearing voices for several years. He said yes, but the hallucinogenic qualities of marijuana could also have caused that. The big surprise for me was having two noted psychiatrists (both well known for work in substance abuse as well as mental health) talk about marijuana being hallucinogenic.

Hunter has been moved from the acute unit to the general psychiatric floor. The purpose is to see how he reacts to increased stress.

The acute unit was very quiet, no groups, and lots of techs. The general unit has an exercise bike, board games, group meetings, etc.

Before release later this week, the psychiatrist will discuss recovery with Hunter. His recommendation is that Hunter stays with us (yes, we are very happy to have him), see Dr. Master weekly, and stay away from marijuana. He will also discuss Hawaii with Hunter and talk about how detrimental it is to him in his recovery.

The hope is that this is cannabis related and that Hunter is disturbed enough by everything that has happened to him that he will stay on his meds and follow a recovery program.

AMEN to that!!

Love,

Mama

Chapter 3

Hunter's mental health crisis affected all of us.

I had no background in the field of mental health. I had no reason to think that I would ever need to have more than a basic understanding of the various illnesses and their effects on individuals and families. My knowledge and understanding were increasing at a fast pace. Unfortunately, firsthand experience was the teacher. I loved being an administrator and teacher in our small school and found that as long as I was actively involved, my mind would not wander into the realm of what-ifs. What if we had recognized the signs of mental illness earlier? What if we had discouraged Hunter from ever going to Hawaii? What if the medicines had worked like we thought they would? I despised the doubting, the wondering if Hunter would ever really be okay. I hated the tears that would roll down my face at the most unexpected times. I prayed with a fervency I didn't realize I had. And I talked with Boo every evening after work. As much as I was trying to process everything that had occurred in such a short period of time, I knew that Michael and Bridget were both struggling to make sense of the past weeks. We emailed back and forth, trying to encourage one another as the days turned into weeks.

In an email to Michael, Bridget wrote:

All I can say is that most family members feel this way when they are dealing with a loved one who's recently been diagnosed with a mental illness. I've been reading up on the illness and the family reaction and I think we've got a nearly "textbook version" of both.

I've spoken to a few people who have family members with bipolar and they live full lives, take their meds and see therapists on a weekly basis. I really think that things will get better once we can get him on the right meds and they kick in. I also think that his having gotten in touch with his spiritual side is a blessing. I find comfort in prayer and I know Hunter does as well.

As far as our work habits—yes, I've been pretty worthless at work. I've been blessed because my supervisors all know what's going on and are being very flexible with me. They've told me more than once that family is my first priority.

I'm also quick to anger and recently I've been crying at the drop of a hat. Marcus tells me that I'm depressing myself and has been very supportive. It's all the emotions and it's all very normal. We need to have a support system for ourselves—Marcus, the church family, each other. If you feel that you're getting depressed or anxious, maybe it wouldn't hurt to start seeing a therapist or possibly find a support group in the area. I know NOVA (and I would think PDX and possibly Lynchburg?) has support groups for families of people with mental illnesses. If nothing else there's AL ANON. Another thing that has helped is actually telling people about it. It may just be me, but I feel a lot better after I talk about what's bothering me.

This doesn't mean that I'm not scared to death. I am very scared for Hunter. I've got my doubts as well, but every time I read through symptoms of bipolar, I know that Hunter is suffering from it. Call it a gut feeling, sisterly intuition, or common sense—whatever—I really believe he's bipolar. I know that it's going to be a rough road, but I know that Hunter would be feeling the same way if it were any one of us. He would be scared but he would do what he thought best. I know he loves us and *appreciates us, even though his mind doesn't realize it at times. He needs us.*

I've prayed more in the past 3 weeks than I did my first 20 years of life. I know that God will see us through this and there is a light at the end of the tunnel. I believe good things happen to good people, and I know that Hunter will get better. Ask and you shall receive.

I love you all.

Love,

Bridget

I thanked God for the blessing of compassion He instilled in our children.

Christmas was upon us. The smell of baking cookies filled the house, along with colorful wrapping paper that needed to be put away. Our Christmas cedar tree, adorned with thirty-years' worth of collected ornaments, sparkled in the living room. Life felt almost normal—except for the fact that as the meds helped Hunter mentally, they also affected his gait, speech, and manual dexterity. His inner clock was off. We could hear him walk a path back and forth upstairs as he tried to use up some of his energy.

We celebrated the new year with grateful spirits and hopes and prayers for better days.

I took Hunter to therapy sessions with Dr. Master in Richmond. He liked and trusted this doctor and felt that he was making progress. During a meeting with Boo and me, Dr. Master stressed patience on our part. We did not want to undermine the progress Hunter was making.

"Having a psychotic break is very stressful for the person involved," Dr. Master told us. "Hunter must have time to reconcile with it. Young people do not often recognize that they have a mental illness and tend to resist taking the meds."

He continued, "Fortunately, Hunter does not fall into the category of denial. He believes that something is wrong with him, and he is willing to do what it takes to heal."

As spring approached, Hunter was physically able to work. He helped our friends the Loys with their vineyard and developed a wonderful rapport with them. Hunter had always been a mix of computer geek and organic farmer, so he put both skills to use by fixing computers and planting an organic vegetable garden. As he grew stronger mentally and physically, he pushed to move out of the house. He was an adult who had lived on his own for years but now felt restricted. Being back in his parents' home chafed him. He wanted to play his music at the volume he preferred. He wanted to cook and eat and have friends over on his schedule, not ours. From winter to spring to summer, we all tried to work through these issues.

A solution presented itself when Bridget and her husband decided to move home. Boo and I had built a new house on the back end of our rural property several years ago and rented our old farmhouse located at the front. The house was now available for Bridget and Marcus. Bridget telecommuted, so they made plans for her to move first. Hunter moved into his old bedroom at the farmhouse shortly after that. This arrangement worked well. High-speed internet was nonexistent in our rural area, but Bridget needed it for work, so she arranged to use it at a friend's house in town. Hunter reconnected with his former horticulture teacher, who had retired, and helped him with various jobs around the house. All my children had loved having Barry Sauls for their ag and horticulture classes in high school. He was one of those teachers who connected with his students and encouraged them to excel in all areas of their lives. Barry lived up the road from us, and Hunter loved visiting him. Watching their heartwarming friendship develop gave me reassurance that Hunter's health was improving—he was expanding his circle of friends and enjoying helping others.

Fall turned to winter, and Marcus still hadn't found a job locally, so he commuted on weekends and holidays to visit Bridget. After many months of sessions, Hunter discontinued therapy with Dr. Master but seemed to do well on his own. His meds had been decreased, and he continued to take them. His physical and mental health seemed to be improving. We watched for red flags but didn't see any. We prayed for continuing improvement and a solid diagnosis. Dr. Master leaned toward bipolar and schizoaffective but couldn't say with certainty that they caused the psychotic breaks. The days passed with a reassuring sameness.

Until they didn't.

A loud *tap, tap, tap* on the back door broke the quiet of our early morning routine as Boo and I prepared to leave for work. *Who would come over this early?* I wondered as I hurried through the house. I felt the same dread that comes with a late-night phone call.

Bridget stood in the freezing air, looking panicked. Immediately, she assured me, "He's okay now."

Alarms went off in my mind as I tried to calm her and listen to what happened.

"I heard banging on the front door a little while ago, and there Hunter was, standing on the porch without a stitch of clothing, shivering from the cold. He told me he was hopping on the roof during the night, but I guess I slept through it. He seems normal now. He's asleep. But you need to know. It scared me to death."

My husband and I were caught between bewilderment and shock as we tried to figure out a course of action. We reluctantly decided that since Bridget said Hunter seemed fine mentally and he was sleeping, we would go to work and call to check on him later. This was not our ideal solution, but it seemed best for that day.

Hunter came by the house after I returned from school and talked with me about what happened. It was a perfectly normal conversation about a perfectly bizarre event.

We sat at our old oak kitchen table, Hunter with his favorite mug of Kona coffee and me with my year-round favorite beverage, ice tea. Without hesitation, he told me his story.

"I remember climbing on the roof, and I wasn't allowed to stay in one place for long, so I had to hop from one part of the roof to the next. Somehow, I ended up on the porch and started banging on the door because I was freezing."

It felt like a dream to him. He was still surprised to realize that it hadn't been. Since he said he felt fine all day and showed no signs of devolving, we called this an episode and prayed that he wouldn't have another one.

The next morning, Hunter found himself under the old oak tree at Bridget's with his arms stretched to the sky, convinced that if he lowered his arms before the sun rose, the world would end.

These delusions frightened Hunter and left him desperate for a good night's sleep. At the same time, he was afraid to go to sleep for fear of waking up outside again.

One morning, I got a call from Bridget on the way to work. "Something isn't right with Hunter. When I woke up, he came into the kitchen, totally ignored me, and grabbed two apples, one red and one green." I clutched the phone tighter and tried to tamp down the sense of panic that was beginning to envelop me. *Oh, God*, I prayed, *please help us. I think Hunter is in trouble again.*

Bridget went on. "He walked past me and out the door with the apples. I started getting ready to drive into town for work, and he came back inside and said some crazy things. Then he went back outside and started tossing the apples to the ground. He picked up the red apple, inspected it, and tossed it away. He did the same thing with the green apple. He kept picking them up, inspecting them, and tossing them to the ground. He's having a break, Mama." The fear in Bridget's voice transmitted easily over the phone and tore at my heart.

Halfway to work, I hit the brakes, turned around, and headed for Bridget's. I called Boo at work and let him know what was going on but that he could stay put, assuming I would be able to persuade Hunter to get in the car so I could take him to the hospital.

Bridget was in the driveway when I arrived. As I stepped out of the car, she ran into my arms, looking for temporary comfort. "Mama," she said with a catch in her voice, "I am so sorry, but I have to go for an important conference call. I don't want to leave you alone, but I have to settle things at work before I can help."

I hugged her and told her not to worry. I felt certain I could handle this and knew I could call Barry Sauls for help if needed. He lived only five minutes away and could be here quickly. As Bridget pulled out of the driveway, I walked up to the house to find my son on the front porch putting his shoes on—first the right one, then the left. He took them off and put them inside the door. He opened the door, took them out, and again put on the right shoe, then the left shoe. I stopped counting how many times he did this.

"Hunter, let's get in the car and go for a ride."

Blank eyes stared at me as he continued to put his shoes on and take them off.

I tamped down a sense of panic and repeated myself.

I finally called Barry, gave him an abridged version of the morning's events, and asked him to help me get Hunter in the car.

He arrived within minutes. Minutes that felt like hours.

"Hey, Hunter," he said. "Let's get in the car with your mom."

Hunter said nothing, then in a flash of movement he sprinted down the hill toward my house.

I ran to my car and headed home. Barry stayed at Bridget's in case Hunter returned.

I took several deep breaths and tried to stop the trembling in my hands as I made the short drive to my house. My mind raced with what-ifs. What if Hunter hadn't gone home? What if he had gone home? What if Hunter continued to deteriorate?

Despite having reassured Bridget that I could handle this, I questioned my inner strength and resolve. I could not even form a coherent prayer beyond *Please, please, please.*

I knew I needed Boo, so I took several precious seconds to call him.

'Boo," I blurted when he answered his work phone, "Hunter is having another break. You need to come home. Now." I hung up before he could respond and prayed he would get home quickly.

Hunter was at the back door with a key in his hand when I pulled up to the house. He couldn't manage to unlock the door, so I took the key and let us both in, desperately hoping I could get him to go with me to the hospital.

We walked into the living room.

"You know the deal, Mom."

"What deal, Hunter?"

"You know it, Mom. I have to kill you and me because the world is going to end. God told me to do this. You have to give me the key to the gun cabinet."

I could hear my heart pounding as I tried to make my mouth form words.

"I don't know where the key is. I can't give it to you."

Oh my gosh, what do I do? The rush of fear from a short time ago took over my entire body and morphed into terror. Who was this person pacing in front of me? He looked like my second-born son, but his actions and words did not fit with the young man I'd raised.

"Yes, you do. You know the deal, Mom. The world is going to end, and I have to kill you and me."

The minutes turned into a quarter of an hour, then a half hour, then an hour, and I heard the same words over and over about the world ending and him needing the key to the gun cabinet.

I made a move to leave the living room, but Hunter took me by the arm and forced me to stay put. How could he be so strong that I couldn't get past him?

I maintained an exterior calm despite my inner panic and continued trying to break through the psychotic haze that had taken over Hunter. He vacillated between agitation and serenity. We even prayed together.

"Our father who art in heaven, hallowed be thy name . . ." The words comforted me and seemed to calm him as well. Hunter was clearly convinced that the world was going to end any minute, and I wanted to ensure that our world did not.

Finally, I came up with something. "Hunter, maybe Daddy put the key under the black metal milk can on the porch." If he checked, he would have to leave the house. "Why don't you see if it's there?"

The minute he stepped outside, I bolted the front door, ran to the back door, and bolted that too. I picked up the phone to call 911. Then the door came crashing in. Hunter reached around me and pulled the phone out of the wall. He grabbed my arm and propelled me into the living room. "Why won't you help me?" he raged with confusion shining in his eyes.

"You know the deal. I have to kill you. The world is going to end."

He reached out and firmly linked out hands together. "Let's pray now," he continued.

Once again, we joined our voices in the Lord's Prayer. I prayed with everything in me that God would deliver us from this nightmare.

Finally, I heard footsteps on the back porch. Boo threw the door open, taking in the destruction and witnessing how bad the situation was.

I wanted to yell at my husband, "Where have you been? I needed you. Hunter needed you." Instead, I tried to tell him what had taken place since I called him at work.

"Dad," Hunter interrupted me. "I need your gun." Again, he rambled about needing to kill us, the world ending, and God telling him to do it. "Mom doesn't know where the key to the gun safe is, but you do."

Boo kept Hunter talking, and I flew up the stairs to the family room, closed the door, and called 911.

I fought to keep the panic out of my voice as I sped through the reason for the call. This was an emergency. Our son was in the midst of a psychotic break and wanted to kill us. We needed help immediately.

Boo's voice wafted up the stairs as he tried to convince Hunter that he didn't need to kill us. Suppose Hunter came after Boo with a knife. Would he have to attack his own son?

I heard footsteps thumping up the stairs. The door flew open. Hunter pulled me by the arm again. I swallowed my panic. Knowing that the police were on their way provided me with a sense of solace, but how long would they take to get here?

"Hunter," Boo said, "let's go outside. It's a beautiful day, and you like being outdoors."

The words fell on deaf ears. Hunter had retreated within his mind again. His vacant eyes told me he was focusing on the words in his head, not on Boo's.

I had noticed earlier that when Hunter wanted us to pray, he calmed down, so I suggested praying again. In the middle of it, Hunter suddenly bolted out the door and off the porch. He threw himself onto the ground and didn't move.

Police cars screeched to a halt in our driveway, and deputies hopped out of their cars.

Spotting Hunter on the ground, they gingerly approached him as Boo and I explained what happened.

"Officer, handcuff me," our son pled as he slowly sat up and offered his wrists to one of the deputies. "I am sick."

The jagged rip in my heart grew larger.

Tears slid down our faces as Boo and I stood side by side, hands entwined, and watched officers gently guide a handcuffed Hunter into the backseat of the police car. Exhausted from the psychosis, Hunter looked at us mournfully through the windows as the car slowly pulled out of the driveway. *Dear Lord, please help this child of mine*, I prayed. *Wrap your arms around him. He is so broken.*

We found ourselves traveling to yet another mental health facility, Crossroads in Fishersville, conversing with yet another staff of medical personnel.

The voices in Hunter's head that we all hoped had permanently gone were back and seemed to speak even louder than before.

Paranoia settled in. Convinced he could read other people's thoughts and they could read his, his mind raced. He awoke during the night too fearful to ask for help. Sleep was a constant struggle, peace elusive.

I made daily calls to Crossroads to check on Hunter and got to know the nurses well. Through watching them, I learned that it takes a special person to work on a mental health floor. I talked with some of the best of those special men and women during Hunter's hospitalizations. The personnel at Crossroads became some of my favorites. No matter what time I called, whoever answered provided me with information and encouragement.

One day a nurse named Marie informed me, "Hunter's day has been difficult for him. He told us that he has been having what he calls 'bad thoughts' most of the day."

She broke the news to me that he'd started having another break but was coming out of it. How long could this continue?

Driving an hour and a half to Fishersville became part of our daily routine. We never knew what to expect when we arrived. When I was in my early teens, my mother and I had a conversation about how life didn't always go as we expected. She spoke words that I still carried with me: "Pray for the best but prepare for the worst." I liked praying for the best outcome, but I had a difficult time accepting the worst. My prayer became, *Lord, help Hunter recover fully, and help me to cope with whatever happens.*

Six days into Hunter's hospitalization, we talked with his weekend doctor. He believed Hunter still heard voices.

"Hunter said his left brain says one thing and his right brain says another. I equate this to good and evil. His brain is fighting itself." Then he told us, "Each time he has a break, brain cells are killed."

The doctor had explained this to Hunter when he'd made his rounds earlier in the day. The revelation that the psychotic breaks killed brain cells frightened him. He didn't want his brain to deteriorate, or to lose his ability to think and reason. He enjoyed intellectual challenges.

The breaks persisted for over a week.

During one update, the nurse told me, "Hunter is having a much better day today. Yesterday he had a full-blown episode and had one-on-one care."

Another included the disheartening news, "Hunter had a total manic trip during the day, which scared him. He was able to participate in groups but was frightened."

Then, "Hunter was having racing thoughts and then felt like he was a robot."

Finally, his nurse reported, "Hunter is doing much better today, not as much paranoia or bad thoughts."

On the home front, emails documented his progress.

Hey Mom and Dad,

Hunter called me a little while ago and we had a good chat. He said it was a rough day, but he was doing better.

Is it just going to be a roller coaster until the drugs get into place? How many days does it take for the drugs take effect?

Love,

Michael

Dear Michael,

Thanks for your email. I'm sure you're feeling a lot better now.

I spoke with the nurse at the hospital and Hunter is doing well. He told them he will stay as long as it takes to get him on the right path. He's asked to be given Seroquel to help him. They have moved him from a level 3 to a level 2, which means we can bring things to him (except chocolate and caffeine). Bridget and I plan to visit tonight, weather permitting. I don't know when he'll be released. You can call him between 12:30 and 1:30 our time, which is just about now.

Talk to you soon.

I love you.

Mama

Thanks for the update. Poor guy stuck in a nightmare! I do wish the meds would hurry up; it hurts to think about him being miserable in this state.

Love,

Michael

Hi Michael,

Mama and I went up yesterday evening. He was still "one on one" with somebody, and we were only allowed to see him individually. Mama saw him first and he wasn't doing that well—very confused and sad that we're only allowed 15 minutes. When I went in, he was doing a bit better. We talked, and he made a couple of jokes about his meds needing to hurry up and kick in. We laughed a bit (which I think is the first time he's laughed since everything that's happened). Anyway, he called me this morning around 8:15 and sounded good—said he'd had a good morning and that they gave him Navane. He thinks the meds are starting to work. He's excited to see Mama and Daddy tonight. I called him around 12:45 this afternoon and he didn't sound that good, didn't seem to be as well as he was this morning but again wanted to see Mama and Daddy. Mama spoke to him around 1:45 or so (I think) and he was hearing voices again and feeling scared, etc.

As of this moment, Mama and Daddy are on their way up to see him again. Unfortunately, I couldn't arrange my work schedule to let me off in time to get up there but am planning on doing so tomorrow.

So . . . that's what I know as of now. Will let you know how tonight went once I talk to them.

Keep praying, he needs it!

Love,

Bridget

Hunter was released after fifteen days. The doctors still had no definitive diagnosis. Some of Hunter's symptoms indicated one mental illness, and some indicated another. His doctors explained that certain behaviors had to be observed over a period of time in order to diagnose effectively. He left the hospital determined to never suffer like that again. He planned to do whatever he could to prevent another psychotic break.

Because of the intensity of his last break, Hunter moved back into his old bedroom at home. He wasn't well enough to hold down a full-time job, but he was able to use his computer skills to work on friends' computers and to work on a website for my school. He also took care of the goats, ducks, and chickens that he had purchased over the past several months. And in keeping with his desire to never have another psychotic break, he attended daily meetings at AA and NA to help him overcome his desire to use marijuana.

About a month after Hunter's release, a local columnist, Dr. Ken West, wrote an amazing story about the pain his family endured because of his father's mental illness. He suggested a law be passed that mandated family members of those with mental illness take a mental health course. As I read his column, I knew I had to share our story with him.

February 21, 2008

Dear Dr. West,

Your column in the Lynchburg News and Advance about your father's psychotic breaks struck a deep chord within me. Our 29-year-old son recently came home after a fifteen-day stay at the Augusta Medical Center's Crossroads. He is currently being treated for schizoaffective disorder/bipolar 1 disorder—according to his doctor, it will take longer to determine a definitive diagnosis . . .

Today, after months of denial, Hunter is convinced that not only does he have a serious mental disorder, but that he also has an addiction to marijuana. He is determined to stay on the medicine regime and participate in the 12-step program of AA. This acceptance on his part and ours has been a gift from God. In this very early phase of recovery, we are all working together to help Hunter achieve maximum health.

The road ahead is long.

Hunter has been to 17 AA meetings in 17 days. His goal is 90 meetings in 90 days. He received his 30-day chip today. We celebrated with a pint of Ben and Jerry's vanilla ice cream. (He has eliminated chocolate and coffee from his diet.)

Like you, we wish we had been able to recognize the early signs of decompensation. And we wish we had acted sooner.

We know now what to look for. We've also been told by the Crossroad's counselor that if we see any abnormal behavior we should immediately contact Hunter's doctor and caseworker. They should be the ones to take action. While it is comforting to have professionals working with us, I pray that if we see signs of an episode we will have the conviction needed to contact these individuals.

Hunter himself has told us what to look for in his behavior. He is terrified of having another episode. Each one causes the burnout of brain cells and that is something he does not want. He still experiences what his doctor calls brain "leaks." His meds are being adjusted to help with this since the first three months after an episode are ones in which further episodes are most likely to occur. It seems that once the brain has experienced several episodes it is easier to succumb to more. Hunter's doctor reminds him that he has a choice with this illness—either he can ride the horse, or the horse can ride him. Hunter wants to ride the horse. My prayer is that he stays on.

For the next several months, Hunter will stay with us. He needs to avoid stress, which is not always easy. He spends his days taking care of his farm animals—chickens, ducks, goats, baby geese, and an incubator filled with chicken eggs. He has also been able to resume some work on a website for Cornerstone Christian Academy, a new Christian school in Appomattox of which I am headmistress.

Medicine and doctor bills are expensive, even at discounted prices, and Hunter has no insurance. Even though Hunter talks about going to work, I wonder who will hire him given his mental illness.

Hunter would like to finish college. He spent seven years at VA Tech and due to what we believe was the unrecognized and self-medicated illness, he still has 24 credit hours of course work left until he will be able to graduate. Again, I wonder. Will VA

Tech ever allow him back given his mental illness and the violence on its campus caused by a mentally ill young man?

That brings me to your suggestion (as I understand it) that legislators make a law requiring family members of the mentally ill to take a course enabling them to recognize impending symptoms of episodes and who to contact. While I agree that we should all know what to look for and from whom we should seek help, I have no faith that the government knows better than we what to do to help our son. A mandated course would be one more stressor for a family already pushed beyond its normal limits. It would also have the probability of creating additional problems. What is the consequence of refusing to attend a course? Jail? A fine? Punish you by placing your child or spouse or parent in a state facility? No, I do not believe that a legislated course is the solution.

Do I think help should be available? Absolutely! I have spent countless hours on the internet researching schizoaffective disorder and bipolar 1. I have learned more about drugs than I ever thought possible. I have picked the brains of every medical professional with whom I have had contact. I would still like to learn more. I would like to take a course that focuses on effective steps to take to prevent death and destruction when the "darkness" falls. I would like to talk with other parents who have had similar experiences. And I would like someone to "fix" our son.

That is God's territory and already he has done quite a bit of "fixing." Hunter believes that prayer is the only thing that got him through the past several weeks. We concur. First and foremost, the Lord kept Hunter and us safe during the episodes. He provided a group of mental health professionals who were able to help all of us. He surrounded us with a church family that lifted us up in prayer. He gave us a family that stayed in contact and offered help. He gave us the strength to carry on when life was very difficult. He moved you to share your very personal story of life with a wonderful father who happened to have bipolar disorder. God is good.

Thank you, Dr. West, for sharing your story. Statistically there must be hundreds who have mental illnesses in the Central Virginia area. Unfortunately, for many of them and their families, they are unable to bear the stigma that the illness carries; they keep their stories hidden.

Our son did nothing to cause his illness. At this time, there is no cure for it. It is simply a life we must all learn to live. With God's grace and mercy, we will.

Sincerely,

Marcie S. Jones

Dr. West's response to my letter was unexpected and filled with understanding.

Dear Marcie,

You are going through an incredible ordeal. And, you are right in my opinion that Hunter will always be on a complicated path. I'm very impressed with your children coming to his aid. Your description of his outbreak (don't know the right word) in your home absolutely hit home. It took me back in time.

I have received a flood of email from people. So, I know you are correct how widespread the experiences your family and my family share are. Many parents and adult children wrote about how they were left out of the counseling process as if they did not exist. That's the part I oppose and hope the state would intervene to help. I think there should be some family therapy offered to family members by attending psychiatrists. And, there should be contact information for emergencies.

But that is another issue. Your story is powerful and moving and continuing. I will keep you, Hunter and your family in my thoughts and prayers. It's a long hard journey and you describe it eloquently. Thank you for taking the time to share your family's story. Very powerful.

Best wishes,

Ken

I had not expected a reply from Dr. West. The fact that he took the time to respond to my letter in such a warm and caring manner comforted me. He truly understood what our family had been through and acknowledged that our journey was not finished.

Chapter 4

J uly 4 promised to be another scorching day in our area.

No worries, I thought. We would have our traditional Fourth of July dinner in our air-conditioned house, and afterward the grandchildren could run under the sprinkler. No fireworks for us, as these same little ones were frightened by the loud noises, so we would celebrate how grateful we were to live in America by waving our flags.

Our country kitchen was filled with the aroma of cooked potatoes and hard-boiled eggs. Mayonnaise and mustard decorated the counter. Celery lay on a paper towel waiting to be chopped. Cubed potatoes drained in a colander in the sink.

Bridget had just dropped off her two oldest to stay with us while she and the baby ran into town for some last-minute items. Running to the store had become one of our Fourth of July traditions. We laughed over it as she headed out the door. I told her, "It isn't the Fourth of July unless one of us has to return to the store for at least one forgotten item."

Five-year-old Etta and three-year-old Hans sat at the old oak table that had once graced their great-great-grandma's kitchen, eating an afternoon snack and chatting with their papa and me. Naturally, the conversation focused on our upcoming evening—savoring chilled watermelon, downing sizzling hamburgers hot off the grill, and running through the sprinkler.

"Gaga," Etta asked, "who's coming again?"

"Who do you think is coming?" I countered.

Etta started naming people: Mama, Daddy, Etta, Hans, baby Sebastian, Papa, Gaga, Uncle Hunter, Aunt Birdie, and Cousin Marylou. Not many compared to years gone by, but plenty considering I was leaving early the next morning with two of my students and a fellow teacher for a conference in San Antonio and hadn't packed yet. I was not typically a procrastinator, so it bothered me that I wasn't ready for the trip. I told Boo to keep the kids entertained while I headed for the closet to at least take out my suitcase before putting the finishing touches on the meal.

The unexpected sounds of a truck pulling into our driveway, a knock on the door, and a strange voice outside sent me hurrying through the kitchen instead. Who would possibly be stopping by at this time of the afternoon on the Fourth?

I didn't recognize the face behind the knock, and before either Boo or I could offer a greeting, the man started talking.

"I just passed a guy on the road. He jumped toward my truck, and I hit the brakes." The story poured out of the stranger's mouth at a frantic speed. "When I asked him what he was doing, he told me he wanted me to run him over."

I gasped.

He kept talking. "I told him he needed help, and I came down here."

My husband and I exchanged looks that told each other we knew exactly who the man was talking about. *It's happening again.*

"Do you know where he is now?" my husband asked.

"He took off across the road," the man replied.

Boo turned to me. "Do you want to go, or do you want me to?"

Thoughts flitted through my mind. *I should go.* I'd been the sole witness to most of Hunter's disintegration. I glanced at Boo and pictured him taking on the memories that I carried.

I grabbed my purse and keys and headed out the door with my husband's words trailing after me.

"I'll call 911."

Chapter 5

"Hunter!"

I hollered my son's name as I came to an abrupt halt in his driveway and jumped out of the car. He'd been staying at his grandma's old house again. He had lived there for about a year before he moved to Hawaii, and he loved the place.

The only sound I heard in the extraordinary stillness of the late afternoon was the trill of the birds. The oppressive heat had sent other wildlife to seek the cooler recesses of the creek. The eerie quiet reminded me of a silent movie and heightened my sense of impending doom.

I spotted the open door of Hunter's old broken-down Honda. My anxiety rose a level. Hunter hadn't been in that car since it breathed its last several months ago. Why would the door be ajar?

Rushing past the vehicle to the back porch, I called my son again. No response.

Despite the emptiness I sensed as I gingerly opened the creaky back door, I continued to call his name.

"Hunter?"

Still no answer.

My eyes took in the scene before me. Kitchen cabinet doors and drawers hung open. Chairs were flipped on their sides. In the dining room, books lay haphazardly about, clothes strewn everywhere.

Glass from the storm door lay on the living room carpet. A fine coating of earth decorated much of the first floor. Overhead lights glared on the destruction, further adding to the spectral scene.

Hunter usually kept a neat home, so this devastation had to be part of a downward spiral. I'd been clinging to the hope that he hadn't deteriorated mentally. That hope was rapidly vanishing.

As I processed the level of destruction, my brain ran the gauntlet from horror to silliness. The oddity of my thoughts disturbed me. *I need to turn out the lights*, my brain insisted. *Boo will be angry that they are all on.*

The house is a mess; I need to clean it up before anyone sees it.

There sure is a lot of dirt for so few plants.

I stopped. How could I even concern myself with these inanities when our son was in serious trouble?

I could not wait to get out of that house. I wanted to leave behind its dankness and destruction. I wanted to walk into the sunshine and see our son standing in the yard with his face lit up in delight. I wanted what I had just seen to be part of an awful dream that I would wake up from at any moment

Instead of rousing myself from a nightmare, I accepted its reality and gingerly stepped off the porch to the front yard. Tamping down the panic in my voice, I again hollered Hunter's name.

And again. And again.

Suddenly, I caught sight of a form moving rapidly in my peripheral vision.

My missing son came loping across our country road like a long-distance runner finishing a difficult race. What he wore—socks but no shoes, cut-off pants, and an open shirt—added to his disheveled appearance. His rapid breathing and wild eyes confirmed that he was present in body only.

As he bent down and picked up both imagined and real items from the sun-browned ground, I wanted to break through his psychosis. Despite knowing that a person experiencing a total psychotic break is incapable of hearing those outside his mind, I still wanted to reach him—to persuade him to come with me. My intellect battled my mother's heart. I needed Hunter to turn back into himself.

"Hunter, let's go see your dad. He and Etta and Hans are waiting for us at the house."

He ignored me.

"Hunter, why don't you go for a ride with me?"

He picked up something only he could see.

"Hunter, hop in the car."

Despite my failure to break through, I continued talking to Hunter, repeating the same statements and witnessing the same results. He acted as if he didn't hear me, his green eyes blank.

Part of me wondered what I planned to do if I broke through the dense haze of his brain and he did get in the car. He could easily jump out while I was driving. Or worse.

Chapter 6

Hunter stared at my Toyota as though it were a mysterious foreign object. I watched him ponder it, standing perfectly still. Suddenly, he hurled himself up from the earth like a gymnast over a vault, crashed his head into the windshield, and bounced off it like the proverbial rubber ball.

I felt rooted to the ground, shocked, unable to process what I had just seen. *This can't be real. Things like this only happen in movies.*

Blood poured down Hunter's face.

He simply stared at me, his eyes as beautiful as ever but looking as if nothing had happened. I cried out his name in anguish.

How could I protect him from himself?

Even as those thoughts raced through my mind, my ears registered the sound of a vehicle coming down the road. Hunter cocked his head toward that same sound. His slight movement triggered panic deep with me.

"No, Hunter. No, Hunter. No, Hunter."

I lost track of how many times I screamed those words.

Oh, God, please help us, I prayed as my son ran toward the road and hurled himself in front of the semi truck, twisting his airborne body upon contact so his spine took the brunt of the hit.

Tires screeched as the driver tried to avoid the unavoidable.

The thud of human on metal and the hum of the truck motor etched itself into my brain.

Chapter 7

Hunter's body sailed into the air and landed with barely a sound on the asphalted road. I waited for him to move. He didn't. Our small piece of earth seemed to hang quietly in anticipation. *Is he alive? Is he dead?*

I was terrified either way.

"Oh my God," moaned the shocked truck driver as he stepped onto the road.

"It's not your fault," I called to him, rushing to my son's side.

Blood gushed from Hunter's head. He stared straight at me.

"I have to stop it. The pain is too much. I have to be with Jesus. It's a million years' worth of pain," he murmured.

Bending as much as my arthritic knees would allow, I cradled his bleeding head in my hands. It looked as if he'd been scalped. Clots of blood seeped onto the road.

Then I heard a *bam!*

Hunter raised his head off the ground as far as he could and tried to slam it back onto the road. He did it again and again and again. Each time I cushioned his head so the back of my hand absorbed the impact. And each time, he told me he had to get rid of the pain—that he had to see Jesus.

My heart cried for my child, but my eyes remained dry. I had to be strong so I could help. Panic was not an option.

When Hunter realized that he couldn't bash his head into the ground, he picked up his hands and tried to choke himself. I didn't have enough arms to restrain him.

I spieled out a litany of family names, telling Hunter that each one of them loved him. "Daddy loves you, Hunter. I love you. Michael loves you. Bridget loves you." On and on I went until I had named all of us in the immediate family. "Etta loves you. Hans loves you. Sebastian loves you. Evelyn and Marcus love you." I ran out of things to say. Television always depicted people saying the most profound things in these situations, but my only desire was that my son know how much we loved and valued him.

It didn't matter if Hunter's thinking was too hazy to understand. I had to say the words. Just in case.

For him.

For me.

Chapter 8

"M a'am?" someone called from the other side of the road. I glanced up and saw the man who had come to our house standing beside his truck. "Ma'am, can I call anyone? 911?"

"Call my husband and tell him to come immediately," I yelled before giving him our home phone number. Whether Hunter lived or died, I wanted his daddy to be able to see him.

I didn't know how much time had passed since the truck hit Hunter. Blood oozed from his head, and foam bubbled from his ears. He was still conscious, and his eyes were filled with agony. God heard a lot from me during those long minutes as I cried to Him. *Oh, God, please help us. I don't know what to do. Please help my son.* Over and over that litany played in my mind as I held my second-born's head and uttered words of reassurance to him.

A siren screamed in the distance. *Someone's coming to help.* A state trooper pulled beside the truck that had hit Hunter. The trooper hurried out of the car and approached me. I have no idea what he said. I only know that I saw his pistol and told him to step back because I believed that if Hunter got a surge of psychotic energy, he would go for the gun in his desire to hurt himself. The officer took my advice without hesitation.

A county deputy had also arrived. He drove his car over the neighbor's grass and onto the road to block the accident scene. No one would be traveling on our road for a while.

"Mama?" My daughter's anguished voice caused me to take my focus off Hunter and the police. There she was across the street. I hadn't heard her van approach, so she must have arrived at the same time as the deputy.

"Mama?" she called again. "Is that Hunter?"

"Yes," I replied, maintaining my sense of calm.

"Can I come over?"

"Yes."

Bridget left the baby in his car seat and crossed the road. Upon seeing her brother, her eyes filled with tears and she started talking to him. Incredibly enough, she reiterated the same words to him that I had spoken earlier: "Hunter, I love you. Daddy loves you. Mama loves you. Michael loves you . . ."

Hunter jerked his hands up to his throat.

"No," we cried to him.

Bridget grabbed his hands and held them by his sides. She once again tried to reassure the brother whose mind was in pieces. "I love you, Hunter. Daddy loves you. Mama loves you. Michael loves you ..."

My sweet daughter lost a piece of herself that afternoon. The piece that connected to her big brother and trusted that he would always be there.

Chapter 9

"We're the paramedics. You need to let us through." I recognized the voice of a dear friend's daughter who, along with her husband, was an EMT. They had heard the report of an accident on their scanner and hopped in their personal truck to rush to our end of the county.

As the trooper listened to Susan identify herself, I echoed her words. "They're paramedics. I know them. They can help."

As soon as the officer nodded his head, Susan and Tom ran to where we were and assessed the accident.

Even some thirty minutes after being hit, Hunter's psychosis, though diminished, was still evident. As Susan gave him a visual once-over, I provided information as quickly and coherently as I could. I started shaking—the impact of the accident had hit me. I needed to maintain my composure to make it through the next minutes and hours, so I took deep breaths and answered questions honestly.

At some point between Bridget's arrival and Susan's appearance, my husband joined us. Upon receiving the call from the stranger who had knocked on our door, he had seat-belted our grandchildren into the pickup and hurried to be with us.

With the arrival of the ambulance, neighbors had started emerging from their houses. One shooed her young son back after coming as close to the scene as law enforcement would permit.

The EMTs put Hunter on a board, placed him in the ambulance, and informed me of their decision to medevac him to the University of Virginia Medical Center. We waited for their helicopter (aptly called

Pegasus) to arrive. In the meantime, the EMTs worked on Hunter in the back of their vehicle, which they had pulled into his yard.

One of the first things they did was give him a shot to calm him down and relieve his pain. They followed that with another assessment and reported his vital signs to the helicopter unit. They kept Boo and me in the loop the whole time.

In the meantime, our three grandchildren were sitting in Bridget's van with air conditioning running, sipping juice boxes and wondering what was going on. Bridget had pulled the vehicle under the shade of a tree at Hunter's house and gone back and forth across the field, first checking on her little ones, then checking on her brother. She repeated that pattern countless times.

With Hunter in the ambulance, Boo and I were also free to check on the children.

Etta looked at me and asked, "Gaga, why do you have mud all over you?"

That was when I realized Hunter's blood had splattered on me. I searched for an answer as Etta peered at me with questioning eyes.

"Gagas get dirty too sometimes."

Etta and Hans burst into laughter. "Gagas get dirty, Hans," Etta repeated. Another peel of children's laughter followed me as I turned to walk back across the field.

"Ma'am, you can't leave until you write down your statement."

My ears heard the statement, but my mind didn't register it. I couldn't imagine being required to detail the events of the afternoon before heading to the hospital to be with my injured son.

"I rushed out of the house so fast that I didn't even take my glasses. I can't see to write anything," I explained to the trooper. *I need to get to my son.*

"Is there anyone who can write the statement for you?" he asked.

Just then I spied Bridget walking toward me.

"Bridget, I have to make a statement before I can leave, and I can't see to write without my glasses. Will you write it for me?"

She took the pen and paper, and I started talking.

"Mama, slow down," she implored after the first few hurried sentences.

"I'm sorry," I replied. "I'll try."

My mind yo-yoed between what had happened in the past hour to what was happening now. How could I provide an accurate account to the police when I could barely concentrate? My mind and heart were with Hunter as he lay behind closed doors in the ambulance. What were the medics doing? Was Hunter still holding his own? Would he make it? With these thoughts and doubts swirling in my head, I abruptly stopped my dictation and rushed through the choppy fields. I needed to see my son, regardless of his condition.

The EMTs allowed me access to him. I awkwardly climbed into the back of the rescue vehicle. Hunter had an oxygen mask over his face and was very still. I knew immediately that he was no longer in the throes of those inner demons. His eyes, though tired with exhaustion, looked clear. He knew who I was and where he was.

Oh, Hunter. My poor, sweet son. I wanted to scoop him up and make him better. But I couldn't. That was up to God.

So I held his hand and reassured him for the few moments I had. Boo joined us and spoke to Hunter, who looked at us with an odd mixture of bewilderment and recognition. His psychosis had passed.

Hunter turned to Susan. "Everything is going to be fine," he told her.

"You're right, Hunter," she replied. "Everything is going to be fine."

This was the Hunter I knew so well. The one who tried to reassure those around him. The one who always saw the bright spots in all of life's challenges.

"Mom, I saw an angel in here," he said. "She was sitting right over there." He pointed to a spot midway up the wall on the other side of the ambulance. "She was beautiful, with long red hair, and had such a serene look. I felt calm just watching her."

He glanced at all of us. "Did you see her?"

I could feel the anxiety level rise in the ambulance as we absorbed what Hunter had just said.

I believed in angels and had listened to Hunter's grandpa tell me about those he saw in the last few weeks of his life. I felt sure of the possibility that an angel had been present, offering solace to our son when he hovered in that misty place between life and death. Part of me wished I had seen her. What an amazing experience it would have been.

"I didn't see her," I finally said. "But I believe you did."

As we awaited the arrival of Pegasus, the rescue team assured us that, despite his injuries, Hunter was strong and responding positively. He was calm and mentally aware, and his vital signs continued to improve after the administration of two bags of fluid. The team medicated and intubated Hunter before the flight so if he had another break, he would be able to breathe.

We heard the helicopter before we saw it. *Thank you, God*, I thought to myself. More help.

The summer grasses swayed as Pegasus landed in the field. The period of calm while awaiting the helicopter was broken as people rushed from rescue vehicle to helicopter and back again. The medical personnel consulted with each other and with my husband and me. A quick squeeze of Hunter's hand, "I love you," and "We'll see you at the hospital" were all we had time for as the team prepared to get back into the air and to the University of Virginia Medical Center as quickly as possible.

As we went through these motions, vehicles stopped on the road, and people climbed out to see what was going on. I didn't blame them for being curious. It wasn't often an influx of emergency vehicles halted traffic or a helicopter set down in a field beside Hunter's house.

I tuned out everything but what had to be done to aid our son. He may have been thirty-five years old, but he was still our child, and he desperately needed help.

Finally, the police allowed the cars to continue to their destinations. We stood there overwhelmed but already discussing what our next actions needed to be. I caught a movement out of the corner of my eye and looked up to see two of our closest friends running across the field. Lynah wrapped me in a warm embrace. She proceeded to offer the same reassuring arms to Bridget and then to Boo. It took me a minute to fully comprehend that she and Rich were standing with us. We had been so immersed in Hunter's accident that we had not contacted anyone.

"How did you know about Hunter?" I asked.

"Susan and Tom called us when they learned who had been hit," Lynah explained. "They didn't know the details, only that it was a serious accident. We left the house immediately. We've been sitting in that line of traffic, too far back to park the car and come to you."

Not only did they rush to be with us, but they also called our pastor and his wife, who were en route to our house.

After talking with Lynah and Rich briefly, we locked up Hunter's house and all four of us headed to our home. Bridget took her little ones to her house farther down the road to clean up and gather what she needed for the imminent trip to the hospital. She also had to call her husband, who was visiting friends in Fredericksburg.

Our pastor and his wife, Geoff and Margaret Hubler, were waiting for us on the back porch. As Boo and I talked about the past hours, I realized I was shaking like a leaf. Shock set in, with hyperventilation holding its hand. My voice hitched as I recalled the events of the afternoon. I forced myself to take deep breaths. Between Boo and me, I think we managed to provide a fairly clear description of the accident for our friends. They listened intently with deep concern in their eyes.

"How can we help?" came from all of them simultaneously.

"Do you want us to drive you to the hospital?"

"Is there anyone you want us to call?"

These questions spurred on the necessary discussion of the next steps—I had to call my parents and contact Susan, the middle school teacher who was going to the conference with my students and me. She would have to go as a solo adult.

Boo had to give his aunt Birdie the news. Birdie was like a grandmother to our children. She'd recently experienced medical issues that caused her to be hospitalized, then transferred into a local health and rehab facility until she was well enough to live on her own. Hunter had been going over to see her several times a day for the past week. He brought her fresh tomatoes and her morning paper, then checked on her house and mail before going back again to visit in the afternoon. We needed to make certain Boo had time to do this before we left for the hospital.

As we bowed our heads for Geoff to lead us in prayer, I glanced down at my feet and was shocked to see my shoes soaked in blood. How did that happen? Then it dawned on me that I'd put my feet and hands under Hunter's head so he could not bang it on the asphalt. My clothes were also sprayed with blood. Etta's earlier comment about the dirt on my face had made me cognizant of blood, but I had not thought about it being anywhere else on me, and no one had mentioned it. Before I did anything else, I needed to shower and change.

As we juxtaposed our desire to start the ninety-minute trip to the hospital with the reality of tasks that needed to be accomplished beforehand, anxiety took root in our hearts. We needed to hurry.

Chapter 10

With three young children in hand, we arrived at the University of Virginia Medical Center. Marcus reached the hospital before we did and managed to find out that Hunter was being prepped for surgery. My mom, two of my brothers and their wives, and three of my nieces had driven to Charlottesville from Richmond and were also waiting for us. Surrounded by this strong support, we made our way to the family waiting area to begin the ordeal that countless others endured in that room—numbering the minutes and hours as someone well loved fought for his life.

I'd never really thought about what a hospital waiting room looked like until this day. The one we sat in seemed pretty standard with its institutional tables and chairs, wall-mounted television set, and an old push-button telephone. Having noticed a bathroom down the hall, we felt set for whatever came next.

Entertaining a five-year-old and three-year-old helped us pass the time. We played games with them, held our sweet youngest grandson, talked as families do, and kept our ears peeled for any news about Hunter. While other family members took turns getting food from the cafeteria, Boo and I couldn't bring ourselves to leave, for fear of missing an update, so they brought food back for us.

As the night wore on, we knew that not everyone could or should maintain the vigil. After our Richmond family left, we decided that Marcus and Bridget should take their van home and leave his car for us. The kids would rest better at home than at the hospital, and Boo and I could drive home in Marcus's car when the time came.

My husband and I spent the long hours that followed in relative quiet. The adrenaline rush of the afternoon had worn off, leaving us emotionally and physically exhausted. We couldn't curl up and sleep but struggled to stay awake as the weight of fatigue threatened to overcome us. Prayer kept us both hopeful and grateful—hopeful for the future and grateful for feeling God's presence as we lived through some of the most difficult moments of being parents. It was during these dark hours that we sent out messages to family, friends, and colleagues.

Bridget and I had already started a Facebook stream to our friends and family, asking for prayer and providing basic information. I wanted the teachers at my small Christian school to hear the story from me, not through the grapevine. I found myself struggling to put the facts and my feelings into words, but I knew it was imperative for me to compose a letter and send it out as quickly as manageable. I began with the stark news of Hunter's psychotic break and continued with details of the accident and the latest update on Hunter's condition.

Hunter is currently in surgery, and as is the case with numerous surgeries, it is taking longer than expected.

As of the last report—two hours ago—his T12 is blown and they are putting pins in his spine to immobilize that portion of the back. The damage is severe enough that the docs are also planning to put pins in the two vertebrates above and below. There is a very real chance of paralysis in his legs. His recovery in the next few days will be a determining factor in the final outcome.

He has a major tear on the back of his skull, but the skull is not broken. Stitching is required for this as well as for his face. We've already been told he may not be as handsome as he was. You can imagine what your face would look like if you had the superhuman strength to throw yourself into a windshield and destroy it!

They've also found a break in his left hand and plan to immobilize it.

Bridget, Boo, the children, and I drove to UVA. Marcus met us there, as did my mom, two brothers and their wives, and three nieces. Etta and Hans have done exceptionally well during this trauma. They know Uncle Hunter was hit by a truck, although Bridget and I are not sure how they acquired that knowledge. Sebastian has also been a trooper throughout the afternoon and evening. Hopefully, they're all getting some kind of rest.

At this point, we haven't heard anything in over two hours. That could be good or bad.

Bridget and I are trying to post updates on Facebook and I will try to keep you updated also.

We have many long days and weeks ahead. I ask the Lord to continue to shower his blessings upon Hunter, his brother and sister, and his dad. I know that God has a plan for all of us, and that as Hunter told Susan, one way or another, it will be fine.

Thank you for your prayers and words of encouragement.

Chapter 11

The surgery continued into the early morning hours. Hunter's medical team called us with updates on his condition as often as possible. The snippets of information gave us hope, despite the length of the surgery. Two hours after I sent the email to my staff, at close to 3:00 a.m. on July 5, we received another update. I immediately sent it out.

Hunter's spinal damage was one of the worst cases the surgeon had ever seen. They put rods in three vertebrae above and below T12. The spinal sac was torn. He bled quite a bit, so they gave him several transfusions. Technically, the surgery went well; however, the extensive damage means that Hunter will be paralyzed from the waist down.

They are currently working on his head wounds. He should be in ICU in a little more than an hour, at which time we will be able to see him for a few minutes. He continues to be intubated and has a cervical collar in case he has stretched a ligament. He will remain fairly sedated for the next two days and will be hospitalized for around seven days. He will have to go to rehab after that to build up his upper body strength and to learn how to cope with paralysis. Bridget and I are both concerned about that. He has walked four miles a day for almost two years and loves being outdoors taking care of his ducks and garden.

The hospital will work with him emotionally, physically, and mentally. They will also work with Boo, Bridget, and me to enable us to help Hunter in the best way possible.

My heart dropped as we continued to receive one piece of bad news after another. I wasn't shocked by the extent of damage to Hunter's body; it just wasn't what I had hoped for. As a person who likes to believe in fairy tales with happy endings, I wanted the prince and princess to live happily ever after. I wanted the miracles in life. I wanted my son to have a body that bounced off the truck without any damage to it.

The reality of hearing an experienced surgeon tell me that my son's case was one of the worst he'd ever seen was more than I could wrap my mind around. What would the ramifications of that be? How would I tell my thirty-five-year-old son, who in his lifetime had already been given diagnoses of autoimmune hepatitis and bipolar, that his spinal cord had been severed and the chances of him walking again were nonexistent? My heart simply hurt.

As the predicted number of hours for the surgery passed, Boo and I shifted our bodies to find comfortable positions in our chairs, quietly waiting for the call confirming the end of surgery. Exhaustion had caught up with us, and Boo was the one who would be driving us home after we saw Hunter. He pushed some chairs together to create a makeshift bed for himself.

As he restlessly dozed, I prepared myself for what the future might hold for our family.

The ringing of the phone jarred us. Finally, we could see Hunter.

Gripping each other's hands, we made our way to trauma ICU, not knowing what to expect, considering the updates from his medical team.

The recovery room was small, filled with monitors, screens, tubes, and wires. The foreign noises of the lifesaving machines shook me. The space was far more daunting than any hospital room I had seen on television. Hunter looked so still and broken lying in the bed, his face covered in blossoming bruises. His head was wrapped in bandages and his neck enclosed in a cervical collar. His bandaged lower right arm lay on a pillow. Tubes protruded from his head and arms. The whole scene felt surreal. Could I touch him?

"You may touch him," the nurse on duty said, as if reading my mind. Boo and I gingerly patted his unbandaged arm. Hunter's eyes opened. He looked at us with deep sadness.

Hold yourself together, I warned myself. *Do not break down now.*

"Hi, honey," I said, forcing my voice past the lump in my throat.

"Hunter Bear," my husband choked out, using his lifelong nickname for our son.

I didn't know what Hunter remembered, if anything, so I told him he had been in an accident and undergone surgery at UVA. He seemed to grasp that even in his grogginess.

"We'll be back tomorrow," my husband told him. "We're going to let you get some sleep."

"I love you," we each told him as his eyelids fluttered shut.

Chapter 12

I knew our family and friends would be waking up soon, wondering about Hunter. While Boo drove us home, I used my iPhone to compose a post-surgery thread on Facebook.

> Boo and I are just leaving UVA. Hunter is in stable condition in trauma ICU. His head has been stitched and he has a couple of drainage tubes in the suture area just in case. His face is also stitched up. He's on meds for pain and sedation. He'll be asleep much of the day, which is good. His progress will determine his departure from ICU—hopefully a couple of days. Then he'll go to acute or intermediate care, and then to rehab.
>
> Boo and I will sleep some and drive back up this afternoon. We ask for continued prayer, especially as we find a way to tell Hunter about the paralysis.

With this message under my belt, I leaned back in my seat and dozed.

Once we arrived home, ever the type A personality, I put a load of clothes into the washer before climbing into bed and falling into a dreamless sleep. I awoke a few hours later, praying for Hunter, for our family, and for me. *Thank you, Lord, for bringing Hunter through this. Please help him to regain clarity of mind. Help his body to heal. Help us to help him as he recovers. Please, God, give me the strength to handle whatever the future holds. Thank you for being with us.*

"With God all things are possible." Those words from Matthew 19:26 (ASV) were inscribed on the silver bangle bracelet that a student had given me years earlier. I wore the bracelet every single day, whether I was at school, church, or home. I had always loved the verse, but today I clung to its truth for dear life. Believing that all things were possible with God had become an anchor, and I needed an anchor more than ever.

After the trauma of the previous day and the long hours spent at the hospital, I was surprised we hadn't slept longer, but the ringing of the phone and the sound of callers leaving messages awoke us. As we struggled to free the fogginess of sleep from our brains, my husband and I fell into conversation about our plans for the day—plans with some flexibility in them since we had never traveled this road before.

Only a few hours had passed since we'd left Hunter, and the nurse said he would be sleeping much of the day, but I still felt compelled to call the nurse's station to check on him. The news that he was in stable condition and still sleeping gave me the comfort I needed, so I placed my next call to Bridget.

She picked up the phone on the first ring.

"We're awake," I said.

She hurled question after question at me, her worry for her brother coming through in her voice.

"I just got off the phone with the hospital, and he's hanging in there," I told her. "Last night was so incredibly long that the minutes seemed to drag on. The quiet was eerie." I shivered at the memory. "The surgical team was wonderful about giving us updates on the operation. I didn't know they did things like that, but I am glad they did. That made it so much easier on your dad and me. We were able to see him for a few minutes after the surgery and talk to his nurses."

As I paused to take a breath, Bridget asked what the nurses said.

Taking a steadying breath, I told her about the titanium rods and pins that Hunter had in his spine—rods that would eventually fuse with his bones to provide a stronger spinal cord for him. I described the sight of his head swathed in bandages. "He has a small brain bleed. On the plus side, his breathing was strong and he seemed cognizant."

Bridget told me that her phone had been ringing off the hook all morning with calls from family and friends. Since we'd also been inundated, we decided Bridget would be the contact person for future calls. I could handle emails and texts, but I didn't have it in me to talk to every friend. I appreciated how much they cared about Hunter, but this crisis had barely begun.

After talking to my mother and Birdie, I called Michael and Evelyn. We had tried to contact our oldest son the previous night, but he was camping with some friends in Oregon, where he lived. His wife couldn't reach him because he was "off the grid," as he called it. Hoping that Evelyn had managed to make contact, we tried again.

"Oh, Marcie," said the sweet voice of our daughter-in-law, "I still can't get him. I am so sorry. I know he is going to be devastated. I've left messages on his voicemail to call me when he gets them. I am hoping to hear from him soon."

While I understood, I was disappointed that we couldn't reach Michael. With one of my children injured so badly, my heart wanted to have the other two close to me, even if that closeness meant hearing a voice from three thousand miles away.

Chapter 13

The afternoon of July 5 brought a barrage of written communication as Bridget and I updated first our family and then our friends.

We're getting ready to go back up to UVA. Hunter is responsive, although still intubated. He will have an IVC—inferno vena cava—today. It will prevent clots from going to the heart, lungs, and brain. The second CT scan, done at 6:30 this morning, showed that a small brain bleed had become even smaller. The hope is to have the intubation tube removed sometime today . . .

Knowing that Boo and I were running on little sleep, Bridget picked us up for the trip to UVA. Silence reined in the van when we drove past the spot where Hunter had lain less than twenty-four hours earlier. I clenched my teeth and took a deep breath to stave off panic. Not too far beyond that place, which the police had marked, we drove right over the line where the truck stopped after hitting our son.

We had driven over this same area yesterday when we went to the hospital and when we came home, but I didn't remember seeing the accident areas marked. Seeing it felt like a sucker punch to my stomach. It had caught Bridget unprepared also.

"I didn't know we were going to see that," she said in a choked voice. "How long do you think that paint will last? It is going to be really hard to drive over it every time we go up the road."

"I don't know," Boo and I replied simultaneously

"I'm with you, Bridget," I continued. "It is going to be very tough to drive over this. It's not like we have another way to get to 460—not without going miles out of the way." One more thing to talk to God about. *Oh, Lord, please help us handle this on a daily basis without falling apart.*

Once we hit 29 North—the fastest route to the hospital—I continued sending updates to family and friends.

Thank you for your calls, offers to come to the hospital, and for coming to the hospital last night. Right now, we simply want to be with Hunter. We will need visits, etc. as time progresses and hope you'll be able to help us then. Starting paperwork for disability and Medicaid Monday. I love you all.

Etta and Hans kept us entertained between email messages.

"Gaga, for Christmas I want Elsa and Anna on ice skates," Etta informed me. She loved everything from the Disney movie *Frozen*.

"Me want Olaf," Hans piped in.

"Well, we'll have to remember to tell Santa when we see him," I told them. "But that won't be for a long time. It's summer now, and Santa comes in the winter."

"That's okay, Gaga," said Etta. "I can wait."

"Me wait too," echoed her little brother.

Talking about Elsa, Anna, and Olaf took my mind off the memory of how Hunter looked when I last saw him. I loved how these two grandchildren of mine could make me smile no matter what was going on.

Driving into the hospital parking garage was as difficult as the evening before, but this time I knew we would be able to talk to Hunter, touch him, and hear his voice.

We checked in with the hospital information desk and put on our visitor ID badges. Bridget stayed in the lobby with the children while Boo and I took the elevator to ICU. Conflicting emotions vied with each other as I walked into Hunter's room: pain over seeing him so damaged, pleasure when I noticed the intubation tube had been removed, gratefulness as I heard his raspy voice, blessed because he was alive.

"Hi, Mom. Hi, Dad," Hunter whispered. "Now, don't cry," he warned us when he saw us struggling to get out a simple hello.

Boo cleared his throat. I reminded myself, *no tears.*

"Tell the truck driver that it wasn't his fault," he told us.

His concern for another even while racked with pain revealed so much about his character. *Oh, Hunter,* I wanted to say. *It wasn't your fault either. Psychotic breaks aren't a choice.* Instead, I reassured him, "I will."

We told Hunter that a lot of people were praying for him.

"I know," he said. "That's the only reason I'm alive. Tell them to keep praying. I think God has a plan for me."

I left the room to trade places with Bridget so she could visit with her brother. After a while, Boo came to the lobby to stay with Sebastian and give me a final few minutes to visit before we left. To our surprise, Etta and Hans were allowed to go with me to see their uncle.

Etta took one look at him, lowered her head, and went to hide behind her mama. She was old enough to be frightened by the change in her uncle. Bridget and I understood her reaction. Uncle Hunter had always been the one to take her by the hand and walk her down to the creek to explain all the wonders of nature. She wasn't used to seeing him bandaged and bruised, lying in a hospital bed. Hans, on the other hand, went right up to Hunter and said hello. His three-year-old mind had no problem adapting to the change.

During this visit, Hunter told us that he couldn't move his legs.

"I think I'm paralyzed," he said with his usual candor.

I didn't know what to say other than he was right.

"Hans," he continued, "I'll take you for a ride in my wheelchair when I get it."

That was Hunter—my child who never held a grudge and tried to find a silver lining in every situation. Riding his oldest nephew on his lap in a wheelchair was the silver lining in this.

Please, God, help us to help our son, I prayed as I listened to Hunter begin the process of reconciling his injuries and his future. *How many times am I going to tamp down tears?* I wondered.

During the drive home, we talked nonstop about our time with Hunter. All three children had fallen asleep within a few minutes of leaving Charlottesville, so we were able to talk without worrying about what little ears would overhear.

We'd left his room as Hunter was being taken for an MRI of his neck, to make sure he had no torn ligaments or broken bones not detected the evening before. I couldn't imagine that he had, given the extensiveness of his surgery, but I was glad the doctors were being so thorough. Until the surgical team cleared him, he couldn't sit up or eat anything other than ice chips. Despite the heavy meds he was on, hunger was gnawing at him when we left. We all empathized with him.

His sense of humor had made us laugh. He told Boo that he would be happy to have a ramp at our house, but he wouldn't be able to help him on the farm anymore. "But," he said, "I can still tell you what to do."

Then he asked for his phone and promptly took a picture of himself to send to his aunts, uncles, and cousins. I rolled my eyes as I read his accompanying text. *Cheers, I'm alive.*

I laughed again, remembering the moment. That was definitely our Hunter.

Chapter 14

The first thing I did on Sunday morning was call the hospital to check on Hunter. The results of the MRI had not come in, but we felt surprisingly calm as we continued to wait. I worried but reminded myself of what our pastor had told us years ago: "Faith is the opposite of fear." I wanted to have faith, so I pushed the fear away and did what I had done so many times in the past—breathed in, breathed out, and said a prayer.

The prayers continued during our church service. At the communion rail, Geoff prayed especially for Hunter. He thanked the Lord for his life and asked for healing. As was his way for those in special circumstances, he anointed Boo and me with oil as he prayed over us. I felt comforted by his words and actions.

The first thing we noticed when we walked through Hunter's hospital room that Sunday was the elevated bed. A surge of joy ran through me. This was progress. He could have more than ice chips now. He had asked Bridget and me to bring him some food so he could eat what he liked when he was able. Now he could enjoy it.

"Hunter," Bridget said as she opened the bag of food. "Look what we brought for you."

His limited mobility prevented him from turning toward her, so we held up the bottles and boxes of broths, fruit juices, and green juices as we placed them in the small cubby in his room. Even with the bruises and swelling, his face reflected his happiness.

"Thank you," our appreciative son said. "Can you pour some of that juice for me now? I am starving."

Bridget immediately poured him a cupful of broth.

My mom and one of my brothers came up from Richmond to see Hunter that day as well. He loved their company but tired quickly. As they talked, I could see the energy draining from him. His eyes closed without warning as he drifted into sleep.

While he slept, Bridget, Boo and I took turns sitting with him. One of us took the kids for a walk around the hospital grounds while the other two stayed in the room, and then we switched places. At Hunter's request, we brought them to his room when he was awake. Once again, Etta tucked her head as she greeted her uncle, but this did not keep her from joining Hans as they examined the noise coming from air compression pumps on Hunter's legs.

"Look, Mommy, I can see Uncle Hunter's legs," Etta exclaimed. "He can walk now."

"Me see them too." Hans pointed to the digital depiction at the base of the air compression pumps.

My heart squeezed over the realization that Etta and Hans thought that their uncle couldn't walk because he had *lost* his legs in the accident. Bridget and I hurried to explain that Hunter's legs were underneath the sheets.

As we prepared to leave Hunter, the nurse came into his room with the results of the MRI from the previous night.

"Mr. Jones," the nurse addressed Hunter. "The MRI showed that your C1 is broken. The neurologist and his team will meet in the morning to determine the best course of action. This also means that you will remain in ICU for a bit longer."

I felt crestfallen as I listened to the report. It was not what I had expected.

Sadness fallowed me home, but I began Monday with a prayer on my lips. *Lord, please help the doctors make wise decisions. Please provide healing for Hunter that will prevent further paralysis. And, Lord, I thank you. The sun is shining, the air is cool, the birds are singing, and Hunter is with us . . . What a wonderful way to begin the week!*

Hunter remained in ICU. He held his own and had a wonderful medical staff working with him. Not quite seventy-two hours after his surgery, he'd already made visible progress. The swelling in his head was going down, the bruising on his face had faded, and his voice sounded much stronger.

Hunter's injuries had motivated me to research the human skeleton and spinal cord injuries. After receiving the MRI results, I turned to the internet to glean whatever information and consolation I could find.

It was humbling to discover how little I remembered from high school and college biology classes about the human body and its intricacies. My research revealed more information about spinal cord injuries than I knew existed, much of it frightening. As a visual person, I searched for articles that offered solid information, reliable organizations, and diagrams of the spinal cord, wanting to understand the exact extent of Hunter's injuries.

I learned that the T12 is part of the thoracic spine, between the cervical and lumbar sections of the spine. The thoracic segments are in the middle of the back. There are twelve of them, and they help control the trunk of the body. I understood that the pins the doctors had inserted into Hunter's spinal cord were necessary to provide support to his damaged spinal cord. I also accepted that his future held many challenges.

I found information on C1 injury (located at the top of the spine) just as intimidating. It could result in total paralysis and the inability to breathe without a respirator.

Years earlier, I'd had a discussion with a parent of one of my students. Her life had taken some unexpected turns, but a specific Bible verse became her mantra. At the time, I understood why she chose Proverbs 3:5–6 (NIV): "Trust in the Lord with all your heart and lean not on your own understanding; in all your ways submit to him and he will make your paths straight." But now I appreciated its comfort in a much deeper way. I had no control over this situation. None. Trusting in God and his plan was my only hope for making it through each day. The verse filled me with courage and strength I could not muster on my own. It gave me an inner peace. And I cherished that feeling.

Chapter 15

It's Tuesday evening, July 8, and I'm staying at the hospital with Hunter.

Lots of news since I last wrote.

Hunter continues to be on several meds—anti-seizure, antibiotic, pain meds, etc.—more than I can remember but fewer than a couple of days ago.

They put in an IVC filter yesterday afternoon. Here is a definition of the process: "An inferior vena cava filter or IVC filter is a small cone-shaped device that is implanted in the inferior vena cava just below the kidneys. The filter is designed to capture an embolism, a blood clot that has broken loose from one of the deep veins in the legs on its way to the heart and lungs."

The neurosurgeon decided not to operate on the C1 but to keep Hunter in a cervical collar. The reason is twofold—one is because the break is minor, and the other is because he's more concerned about pulled ligaments. We need our neck ligaments to support our heads, and it seems that Hunter's are damaged. The Dr. has ordered an x-ray of the neck while Hunter is in the Stryker chair at a sixty percent incline.

Hunter was moved from ICU to acute care late yesterday afternoon. While the medical staff is good, there's not as much one *on one. I got a phone call at 6:00 this morning from Hunter. He couldn't get the nurse, so he asked me to call them to tell them he needed help. That's when we realized it would be helpful to have one of us with him.*

An ultrasound of his legs showed no clots, and blood work revealed no Hep C. The bandage on his head will be removed tomorrow. He is also scheduled for surgery on his hand, and yes, it is his right one. I got it wrong in my earlier email. He broke a joint in his middle finger and it needs to be repaired.

Hunter sat up for the first time today. His nurses, PT, and nurse practitioner were all impressed with how well he did. Hunter said it made him feel like he had successfully completed a parachute jump.

Still not clear on a timeline—I've tried to catch up with the social worker to no avail. I'll work on that again tomorrow.

Michael and Evelyn fly in on Friday morning. All of us are looking forward to seeing them.

Please continue to pray without ceasing.

This email to my family provided them with the latest facts on Hunter but not the inner turmoil I felt after that 6:00 a.m. phone call from him. It felt like a kick in the gut.

My heart had dropped when I heard his frightened, tearful voice plead with me, "Mom, please call the nurse to help me."

I could only imagine the depth of fear and despair he must have felt. He couldn't get anyone to reply to his calls for help. He was paralyzed and in pain with his head in a cervical collar and his right hand covered in thick bandages. He depended on others, and for whatever reason— not enough nurses, too many patients, someone else in need—help hadn't arrived.

"Try to calm down," I'd assured him. "I'll call the nurse's station and get help for you. And I'll be at the hospital as soon as I can get there."

Boo and I talked about that emotional phone call and realized that Hunter needed someone with him for the duration of his hospital stay.

"I could hear the panic in his voice," I explained to my husband. "This isn't like the ICU where he had constant supervision. He's alone and he's frightened."

"You're right," he replied. "He needs someone with him to help him, but I can't be there during the week because of work."

"I know you can't, but I can. I can pack a bag and take my computer with me to do schoolwork. I'll have my phone, and I can always contact the principal or admin if there's something I need help with." The beginning of July was typically a slow time for us, so I didn't anticipate issues.

My heart felt wrung out like a twisted washcloth. I not only wanted to be the one to go to Hunter, I needed to be the one to go to him.

Sensing this, Boo held me in his arms a bit longer than normal before he left for work. "Call me when you get there."

Chapter 16

"We're going to put you in the Stryker chair, Mr. Jones," one of the physical therapists told Hunter.

"Okay, let's do it," he answered. "What do you want me to do?"

"We'll talk you through it," the PT assured him.

I almost asked what a Stryker chair was but didn't want to interrupt the physical therapy session. The idea of him moving to a chair of any kind concerned me.

Three days earlier, Hunter had lain unconscious in ICU with titanium pins and rods in his spine. Now they expected him to sit in a chair? Good grief! What were they thinking? How could they move him? His neck might break. His sutures might leak. His spine might fracture more.

These thoughts ran haphazardly through my brain as I watched, with great trepidation, the two therapists move Hunter from the hospital bed to the chair. The process of moving him took some time, but as I watched their precise but gentle movements, I felt confident these therapists knew what they were doing. I had never realized how physically challenging a physical therapist's work could be. One of them had to kneel on the bed to help hold Hunter upright while the other held the sheet, which they used as a type of pulley to get him from horizontal to vertical. Then they had to get him from the bed to the Stryker chair—a thick-cushioned type of recliner that supported both the body and the head.

"Take pictures, Mom," Hunter instructed me. He wanted photos of every part of his recovery.

Curious by nature, he liked to share his experiences with others. He had been known to catch bees between his thumb and index finger and show them to Etta and Hans, explaining the anatomy of the insect. Now he hoped others would learn from his experience with physical therapy.

"Okay." I shook my head in wonder and slipped away.

His face revealed the concentration and effort it took to move from bed to chair. Under any other circumstances, he would've smiled at his accomplishment. But he was in such pain and had so many abrasions on his face that he looked like what he was—a young man who had been hit by a truck.

That first full day at the hospital was packed with activity. Our son Michael had returned from his hiking trip to face the trauma of his brother's accident. Sending emails and texts to him, his wife, Evelyn, and Bridget and Boo had become as routine as feeding the animals.

Hunter sat in a Stryker chair today. The PT said he did a remarkable job with his first time up. He'll spend an hour in the chair today and work himself up to three two-hour periods over next couple of days. Physical therapy wore him out, but he said it was an amazing feeling to sit up.

Michael immediately replied:

Good to hear! Sounds like a strong start on the road to recovery!

I wrote back:

I think it is. He's in pain now and waiting for his meds. He has a high tolerance for pain so I know he is hurting when he starts taking deep breaths. The Neuro doc just came in and said there was some minor seepage from Hunter's back, but it is okay. X-rays of neck with him sitting up will happen shortly. Dr. is concerned about pulled neck ligaments more than fractured C1. The collar will be on for at least two months.

Ligaments support head so the healing is very important. No blood clots in legs, no Hep c, and removal of head bandage tomorrow Hunter requested 5 mg of meds due to pain and is sleeping. Busy afternoon.

I barely slept that night. I curled up in a cushioned window seat with a pillow and blanket, trying to find a way to get my less-than-compact body into a comfortable sleeping position. My battle with sleep was nothing compared to Hunter's.

We had a terrible night. Hunter worried about the upcoming hand surgery and the neck x-ray, so he got very little sleep. Between the anxiety, lack of sleep, and pain, he said things that sent my antenna up.

"I have to get away. They can hear everything."

"It's okay, Hunter," I told him as I walked over to him.

"You don't understand. I have to get away."

I recognized these beginning signs of a mental episode and immediately went to get a nurse. I wanted her to give Hunter an Ativan for anxiety immediately, but she couldn't do it without a doctor's permission, and the doctor had to talk to Hunter before prescribing it. I knew this was protocol, but I was so worried that I wished they would just do what I said.

Finally, the prescription came through. After Hunter took the Ativan, his anxiety level decreased enough for him to fall into a fitful sleep.

Before I dozed off, I emailed friends and family and asked them to pray along with me.

Please, Lord, watch over my son. Guard him and protect him. Give him a sleep free from this awful pain. Help him as he enters surgery.

When I checked my email later in the morning, I grew teary eyed as I read messages of encouragement in response to my request. The first one was from my niece Frances.

Hang in there. I can't imagine how hard this is. Just know there are lots of people praying for you all! Mental illness is . . . I can't even think of a word for it. Just know that I understand. I love you.

My sister Sally wrote:

Thanks, Marcie, for your updates. Yes, praying for Hunter and his surgery today. Praying for the surgeons and all of the staff at the hospital working with Hunter, that they will be divinely guided to do their best work. Praying for you, Marcie, that through all of this tragic last few days you are able to get some sleep, some direction as to what needs to happen and when, and some moments to yourself to regroup. Please stay aware of your own health during this extremely stressful time. I am so thankful that you have such a solid prayer life and relationship with God. Hunter is such a remarkable man, and you have instilled in him a strong sense of resilience, which is evident especially over the last few days. I love you, Marcie. Call whenever you want to.

At many times throughout my life, I had talked with people about how a crisis could either bring a family together or tear it apart. While my extended family had had its share of challenges, this one seemed to top the list. The love and support from all of them confirmed my hope and belief that we would survive this trauma.

Chapter 17

I learned quickly that, except for a few hours in the very early morning, hospitals are not quiet places. Patients in Hunter's condition required a great deal of help in the recovery process. He had to be turned every two hours or so to prevent bedsores, and though he would learn to do this himself as he progressed, at this point he needed nurses to do it for him. They were working around tubes and IV machines, as well as the neck brace and the special apparatus on his legs that alternately applied and released pressure. Not to mention the care they had to take due to the pins in his back and the accompanying slice on his spinal cord.

The schedule for the meds and the vital signs continued 24/7. Specialists checked on Hunter according to their own schedules, even if it was 4:00 a.m. The day of his hand surgery was no exception. As usual, each resident and member of the surgery team was caring, courteous, and knowledgeable. They took time to talk with Hunter and answer his questions, which he recorded on his iPhone as soon as they popped into his mind. I was relieved to see that even after such a severe head injury, his intellect seemed perfectly intact.

The anxiety Hunter had experienced the night before meant that neither of us slept well. The Ativan helped his anxiety immensely, but his pain level had increased and his IV was leaking. I went to the desk to ask a nurse to check on it. She replaced the IV and gave him more pain meds. That medicine helped him manage his pain for the next few hours as he awaited surgery, which was scheduled for 1:30 p.m.

Hunter groaned.

I put my hand on his arm. "Are you still in pain?"

"No. I'm starving."

I looked at my watch. He still had hours to wait for food. Soon it would be lunchtime and Hunter would have to smell the evidence of it. "I'm sorry, honey. I know this is hard."

When the hospital attendants finally appeared at the door to take Hunter to surgery, we both let out a sigh of relief. This was a minor surgery compared to what he had already endured, but we still felt stressed over it. The rapid beating of my heart and dryness in my mouth reminded me that one of my babies was being wheeled out of the room for another surgery. I walked as far with him as the medical team allowed and staved off tears as I reassured him that everything would be fine.

"I love you," I said when I reached the point where we had to say goodbye.

"Love you too," he replied in a husky voice.

Taking a walk outside the hospital was the best thing I could do for myself while waiting. Despite the heat and humidity of the day, I needed to be outdoors and pretend everything was normal. During this venture, I discovered my favorite place in the medical center: the quiet area outside the cafeteria. I smiled as I watched the small birds flit from one dropped breadcrumb to another. I admired the vivid colors of the flowering plants. I marveled at the quick pace hospital personnel kept as they clipped their way across the courtyard. I breathed in deeply, then out. I said a prayer. *Thank you, God.*

Not long after that, I returned to Hunter's room, and the techs wheeled him in. The surgery on his middle finger had gone well. The doctor had repaired the torn ligament on his finger and the break above the knuckle, then splinted his hand. The plan was to replace the awkwardly large hand splint with a smaller finger splint in a few weeks.

"I didn't realize the splint would be this big," Hunter said as he turned his hand over to gauge the size of the entire bandage.

"I didn't either." I looked it over too. "I know the break was bad and that the damage to the ligament concerned the doctor. I expect the bandage will prevent any damage if you accidentally knock your hand."

Hunter gave me an exasperated look that I could easily translate. *Really, Mom,* his eyes relayed, *there is no way I am going to accidentally hit this hand.*

My response got put on hold when a doctor I didn't recognize walked into the room. Since the surgery had not required sedation, an eye exam had been ordered. After dilating the eyes to rule out damage, the doctor gave Hunter an all-clear diagnosis. He also let us know that the ugly clot in Hunter's left eye would disappear in a few weeks. Relief poured through me, and I sent up a prayer of thanks.

As Hunter tried to get some rest in the late afternoon, I sent an email to family members.

Hope you're all doing well. Hunter is in more pain now than other days. He still does not want visitors, as it is hard to cope with pain and visit. I am working on disability and Medicaid. At this point, he'll be in the hospital another seven days. He will go from here to rehab—still hoping for UVA. Please continue to pray as we enter different stages of recovery. The challenges are immense but absolutely surmountable.

Whenever the nurses or doctors came in, they asked Hunter about his pain level. He never put it higher than a six or six and a half. I decided that he had inherited my mother's high tolerance for pain, because his stifled moans and anguished expressions indicated a pain level of ten. When his pain got worse, his good nature showed signs of irritability.

As he sat up in bed to eat his first solid meal in a week, he lamented that he was getting full quickly. I reassured him it was probably because this was his first real meal since the accident

"It wasn't an accident, Mom. I ran in front of two trucks and choked myself. I tried to kill myself. Call it what it is."

I didn't bother to tell him that he was in the throes of a psychotic break and wasn't thinking straight when it happened. He wasn't in a frame of mind to hear that. He was intent upon being his own judge and jury and had found himself guilty.

With a deep sorrow in my heart, I recounted this to my sisters, who had all been sending me private messages.

It was a decent night considering we're in a hospital and the nurses and techs come in every two hours for body rotations etc. Hunter is in a lot of pain. He's afraid he'll become addicted to pain meds. The doctor said he would be on them for three or four weeks. He told his nurse that he thought his body was becoming used to the meds, and she told him that wasn't true and he needed to take them to help his body heal. That seemed to reassure him. He just took another dose and should get some sleep.

I appreciate the good thoughts and prayers.

I love you all.

Chapter 18

By Thursday, July 10, it felt like forever since Hunter's accident, but it had not even been a week. Bridget made the trip to the hospital with the children every day. Even with work, the farm, and visiting his aunt in the health care facility, Boo made it a priority to come every other day. Some days he rode with Bridget and the kids; other days he headed straight for the hospital from work.

"Gaga," Etta greeted me on one of those visits, "Uncle Michael and Auntie Evelyn are coming!"

"They are?" I asked, pretending not to know. "How wonderful."

"When will they get here?" Hunter asked.

"They'll be here tomorrow," Boo answered him. "They found a hotel in Charlottesville and will stay there for a couple nights. Evelyn has to return sooner than Michael, so it was better for them to stay here. Michael will spend his last night at the house before he has to fly back."

"Their hotel room has a pool," Bridget added. "Evelyn said she'd take the kids for a swim while we visit with you, Hunter."

"They'll like that," he responded.

Listening to the conversation, all I could think was how blessed I felt to have all my babies together again.

When they left later that evening, I walked them to the parking garage.

Boo expressed concern that I was wearing myself down staying at the hospital day and night.

"I've emailed Michael about staying a night with Hunter so you can come home and get some rest. He is more than willing to do that, and it will be good for Hunter and him to have some time together."

"They're taking a red-eye here," I told him. "Michael's going to be physically exhausted when they arrive, and seeing Hunter for the first time will be emotionally challenging. Staying the night will only add to his fatigue."

"He can handle it, Marcie," my husband assured me.

"I know he can, but it is going to be hard for him."

My Facebook update related some of the day's events:

Hunter continues to improve daily. He can sit up and move himself to either side. He does have leakage from the spine, which is of enough concern to the surgeons that another MRI was done this afternoon. We hope to have results of that in the morning. Of course, we would like to hear good news. He is in a lot of pain but does not complain at all. His positive attitude and willingness to do whatever it takes to help him recover to the highest level possible are such blessings. The medical staff has commented numerous times that these characteristics will help him immensely as he faces the many challenges ahead. Hunter is looking forward to seeing his older brother and sister-in-law tomorrow. All three of our children will again be together—a miracle in itself. Your prayers for his recovery are truly appreciated. We ask you to keep offering them up. God continues to work in our lives daily. Many have asked about visiting. At this point, it is too much of a struggle for Hunter. I'll let you know when that changes.

Morning found Hunter anxious to see Michael and Evelyn, but life in the hospital went on regardless of who was coming.

During his daily morning visit, Hunter's surgeon reported that his latest MRI confirmed spinal fluid leakage. "But since it has slowed down, we're going to continue to bandage it rather than consider surgery," he explained.

Chapter 11

"That's good," Hunter told him. "No offense, but I don't want another surgery."

"If you maintain this progress," the doctor continued, "you could be released sometime after Monday."

I couldn't believe what he had just said. Of course, we had to wait for a rehab center to be confirmed, but Hunter was doing well enough to leave the hospital in just a few days. *Thank you, Lord!*

Brimming with this good news, Hunter asked the nurses to help him into the Stryker chair to wait for Boo to bring Michael and Evelyn from the airport. Bridget had coordinated with her daddy about the expected arrival time so she and the children could be at the hospital when they arrived.

When Michael finally walked through the door, I smiled through my tears as brother welcomed brother. Being careful to touch only Hunter's shoulders, Michael gave him a squeeze. Evelyn leaned in for a peck on the cheek. With the appearance of Bridget, Etta, Hans, and Sebastian, my world felt complete.

To have all three of my children together again was our belated Fourth of July miracle. They spent some sibling time together while Boo and I stayed with the grandchildren in the lobby. Later, Evelyn took Etta and Hans to the hotel pool, which proved to be the perfect distraction from the reality of the hospital. Just as Michael and Hunter were great uncles, Evelyn was a wonderful auntie. She loved children and had the gift of making them feel like they were the most important people in the world. In return, Etta and Hans adored her.

When Evelyn rejoined us at the hospital later in the day, she regaled us with stories and photos of the afternoon's adventures. By now, Hunter was noticeably hurting. The doctors and nurses had continued to reassure him that he was not taking enough oxycodone to become addicted, but he still worried about it and took less than he needed to control his pain. Despite this, he still managed a smile at the images of the little swimmers. My heart filled with a bittersweet admiration at his determination to remain positive regardless of how he felt.

Chapter 19

The time with Michael and Evelyn helped all of us. I spent two nights at home while Michael stayed with Hunter. I was able to catch up on some household chores, recharge, and to simply be.

By this time, Hunter was sending his own emails. He was still concerned about becoming addicted to the pain meds after overcoming a drug problem already. When I read the email he sent to Bridget on the second night of Michael's stay, I wanted to cry all over again.

The pain meds r drastically affecting my thoughts.

  right now I am waiting for them to kick in to sleep some b4 the 2 hour rotation.

  I have clear simple thoughts during this next 15-35 min, when pain relief is being increased and loopy side effects kick in

  pls share this with dad mj n mom

  pain from various healing parts

  hand stomach back area

  pain from neck brace location

  head pains

Michael's email offered information on his observations and on the doctor's report.

Really good night of sleep (for both of us). Numerous blocks of 2hr rest.

IV unplugged means no stupid buzzer. Also pain mgmt. is better.

The neurosurgeon said x-rays looked great. Said they lined things up as best they could, and things will grow over time. He can expect to regain feeling over months & years. I asked if he meant complete or incomplete. Neuro guy said complete, so Hunter knows he is "t12 complete." Hunter seems to be doing a lot more thinking about long-term implications . . . I hope there is counseling in rehab. He wanted a thermometer to measure temp of his legs. I talked him out of additional gadgets. He's ok using his hand to sense temp by touch. Last night was 10x better than the prior night.

Michael and I traded places that Sunday afternoon. He took Evelyn to the airport and drove back to our home in Spout Spring. Before he and Evelyn left, they talked with Hunter about an idea they'd already shared with Boo and me.

"Evelyn and I have been talking," Michael told his brother. "We want you to consider coming to live with us. We think we can remodel the bottom floor so you can have a small efficiency with ground access."

"Are you serious?" Tears choked Hunter's voice. "You really think you can do this?"

"We're going to try," his brother replied. "It will take some time to get everything pulled together, so you will be at Mom and Dad's until then, but we think it can happen."

If this worked out, Hunter would have more opportunities than we could hope to provide for him. If it didn't, then I knew God had something else in his plans.

I once again took up residence in Hunter's room and updated my family.

Hunter got into the wheelchair for the first time today. He's doing an amazing job—even turned a 360. The pain is less when he is sitting rather than laying down so that's an added benefit of the wheel chair.

I smiled to myself as I wrote those sentences. I had never given any thought to how paraplegics moved from bed to chair and back. I watched intently as the physical therapists instructed Hunter on how to use a sliding board to scoot himself from the bed to the wheelchair. Hunter responded perfectly to each detail and made slow but steady progress. His determination to succeed was rewarded with every inch of movement.

I held my breath as I watched him lift himself and make the final slide from bed to chair. I heard him express fear that he might fall, and I privately feared the same thing. The well-trained and empathetic therapists assured him that they would not let that happen. Hunter's joy at being able to move himself around the room sent tears rolling down my cheeks. His laughter as he spun in a circle made me smile with pride.

"Look at this, Mom," he said, eyes alight with joy as he wheeled himself around. "I can't wait to show Daddy and Bridget. They don't know anything about this. I bet Hans is going to love taking a spin down the hall with me."

Later, I sent another update.

Bruises continue to fade and bones to heal. The cervical collar will remain on for 6-7 weeks due to the pulled neck ligaments as much as the fractured C1. The spinal fluid leak lessens daily. Hunter can move himself from side to side without aid now and can lift himself up from the wheelchair every half hour as required. Since he can't feel his lower body, the lifting is necessary to prevent bedsores. I don't know when they remove the staples from his head and his back . . .

Short and long-term plans for Hunter include going from hospital to rehab to Spout to Portland. They're talking four to six weeks in rehab (which has been described as a boot camp), a couple of months with us, then on to Michael and Evelyn's. Michael and Evelyn are hoping to have their bottom level (street level) floor converted into an apartment for Hunter. Portland is ranked #5 in the nation for livability for people using wheelchairs. Hunter will have family, high-tech availability, job opportunity, socialization, and so much more. As a mom, my heart hurts to have another child so far away but rejoices that the new home is one of such opportunity on all levels and will bring two of my children together. God is good!

Thank you for the ongoing prayers. As Hunter just said, "That's all it is, the prayers." The road to recovery is just beginning and like all roads, there will be twists, turns, and bumps. I pray for the Spirit to guide us as we make our way into the future.

With love,

Marcie

Lynah was one of the first to reply.

Oh my sweet friend. I have been so worried about you and am happy to hear that you were able to sleep in your own bed for a couple of nights. You have always been a remarkable woman in my eyes but even more so now. You faith is incredible and such an inspiration to all of us who know you. Michael and Evelyn are a blessing to do all this for Hunter's future. The relationship among all of you is one of the reasons I fell in love with your family all those years ago.

Chapter 20

Back at home, my administrative assistant, Teri Houts, had set up a meal train for our family. She knew that Bridget and Boo were traveling to Charlottesville almost on a daily basis and that having meals brought to the house would help eliminate some stress.

In our community, one of the first things we did when people suffered a severe trauma or lost a family member was to take food to the household. Offering prayers and preparing meals were sometimes the only comfort and aid we could give our friends. I had done this for years because I wanted to, but I had never considered how much it meant to the family in need. I learned firsthand how much these meals could help in a crisis.

"Stacy Hackett and Lisa Fetty brought dinner last night, Mama," Bridget told me when she and the kids came to visit Hunter. "You should have seen Daddy eat that ham! It was so good that he had two helpings. Even Etta and Hans gobbled it down. They also brought coleslaw and potato salad."

"That's great," I told her. "That means your dad was able to pack leftovers for his lunch. I know that made him happy. I'm pretty sure he hasn't had time to go to the grocery store to shop for any kind of food, much less to make a special trip for lunch items."

"That's exactly what he did," replied our daughter. "There was actually enough for all of us to eat supper last night and have lunch today. It was great."

Bridget's face lit up. "I meant to tell you that Mrs. Van Noordt made the best rolls and cream puffs and sent them to us. I mean, they were seriously delicious. You need to get the cream puff recipe from her. I'll make some if you do."

"Is that your way of telling me that you all ate every last cream puff?" I teased.

"Well, we left some for lunch for Daddy and Etta and Hans, but they really were hard to resist." My daughter had a twinkle in her eye. "Oh, and did I mention that the Hublers said they were bringing Indian food and that Cynthia Spiggle called to see what everyone liked to eat?"

"No, you didn't." I knew how much the family loved these specialty foods and was grateful that our friends were making such an effort to prepare unique dishes. "I know that is going to be one delicious meal. Do you think you can bring some leftovers to me?" I joked.

"I'll make sure we leave some for you," Bridget promised.

I had always been glad that everyone in our family could cook. But being able to cook and finding the time to do it were two different things. Boo and Bridget could have made it through on their own, but the meal train made it so they didn't have to. I didn't need to spend a minute wondering if they were taking time to eat properly. We were all able to focus our time and energy on what mattered the most at that point—helping Hunter to heal so he could come home.

Chapter 21

As Hunter and I again settled into a hospital routine, we learned the extent of his limitations and strengths. He had to do everything from tooth brushing to using his phone to trying to dress himself one handed. It was even a challenge to reach for the box of tissues, because he had little balance due to the paralysis. Sometimes I got up and down from my chair a dozen times in an hour to retrieve something that fell or was out of Hunter's reach.

"Crap," he snapped one day. "I can't even get a tissue out of the box without starting to fall over sideways!"

"I'm sorry," I said. "I know this is hard, but look how far you've come in such a short period of time."

"That's not good enough," he retorted.

There was nothing I could say that would help. I fell back on my habit of praying when I faced a seemingly impossible situation. *Lord, please help Hunter cope with his loss. Give him patience with himself. Please help me to help him.*

The possibility that Hunter might have another psychotic episode was never far from the surface of my mind. He seemed to be doing well, but stress was one of the precursors to a break, and he was definitely stressed. At the same time, I saw no red flags.

Mornings were when doctors stopped in the room to check on Hunter's progress. Usually, they had all come and gone by breakfast. They checked the sutures in his back and head, examined his neck and legs, and read the nurses' reports. They asked about his pain level and talked about what the immediate and long-range future may hold.

On some days, the regular surgeons visited and the rehab doctors also stopped by to introduce themselves and discuss their part in Hunter's recovery.

Physical and occupational therapists continued their work at various times of the day. I gave up on figuring out exactly when to expect them. Most of the therapists were amazing. But on two separate occasions, a therapist came into the room, introduced herself, and proceeded to tell us that she was there to help Hunter walk. I couldn't believe what I was hearing.

"Excuse me?" I questioned the first therapist, thinking I must not have heard correctly.

"I'm here to help Mr. Jones walk," she repeated.

"He can't walk," I told her. "He's paralyzed. His spinal cord is severed." I couldn't think of any words to sugarcoat Hunter's condition.

"I'm sorry," she said. "We'll do something else."

I bet you will, I thought, restraining my urge to ask if she had read Hunter's chart.

Hunter shook his head and asked what she needed him to do.

I started the paperwork for Medicaid and disability and found the process slow, discouraging, and overwhelming. I considered myself intelligent, but my master's degree was of no use as I tried to maneuver my way through the system. I found myself wondering how others figured out the correct steps. The hospital had people available to help with the paperwork, but it was difficult to make the needed connections. The Fourth of July weekend had thrown everything behind, and Hunter was not the only one who needed help. I made calls to the hospital office and finally decided that the best thing to do was put a face to the voice on the phone by visiting the office. After several tries, I reached someone who could move the process along. I was thrilled. Social workers started showing up to ask Hunter and me questions. I felt befuddled by it all, but they made everything seem easy. Relief flooded me as the necessary documentation made its way to the proper authorities. Another *Thank you, Lord*, moment for me.

Hunter and I continued to sleep sporadically, so I updated folks at all hours of the day and night. Michael and Bridget were always available for texting with me, and I didn't hesitate to communicate with them regardless of the time. I knew they would reply when they could.

Not much sleep at all last night—actually, it was the worst yet. He is simply not sleeping except for small periods of time. Neuro and trauma have been here. Trauma is quite impressed with his recovery; neuro said back looks good. Head neuro doc should be in soon. Collar pad to help with discomfort. Emotionally, he's all over the board—goes from treating me like an idiot to thanking me for my help to cursing at little things. I am praying my way through this.

Hilarious—Hunter just told nurse he'd gotten more sleep last night than ever!

I didn't filter a lot of what I wrote to Michael and Bridget, but I gave the less-detailed version to our Facebook friends.

Hunter continues to make great progress. He can turn himself in the bed and get himself into a wheel chair with minimal help. He greets the nurses, doctors, and patient assistants with a warm, "How are you doing?" He even has some of them chuckling with his banter as they give him shots in his stomach or help in some other way. The doctor removed some of the staples from his head and back today with the promise to remove the others in a few days. He now has a custom brace on his right hand so that he will not injure his hand any further as he tries to move himself. We're still waiting to learn where rehab will take place and I ask for your prayers as we approach this next step. God has been so good to us and I pray that His hand will be with Hunter as we find a rehab facility that can provide the most help to him.

And in yet another family email, I provided further updates.

Below are the notes I took this morning from the doctor who talked with Hunter. She is a liaison between UVA and HealthSouth.

July 16, 2014

A new doctor visited today to do another evaluation. Notes are below.

Trying to get Hunter into rehab at UVA—calling his doctor to talk with him about this

High tone, Low tone in legs—need to read about this

Bulbo cavanosous reflex—feel for contraction of anal sphincter—first reflex to return after injury—tells whether suppositories will be effective

Need to protect skin particularly skin around bone

Safest thing found is to prop pillows under one side of back when turning

Pressure release mattress is necessary for bed

If in a good pressure release mattress, can stay on longer period of time without skin breakdown

Portland—find a good spinal cord injury doctor

Will be on blood thinners for a while (heparin now)—about three months—will take out clot catcher at about six months

Currently in catabolic state—coming out of it—but burning lots of calories—may prefer to eat small, more frequent meals

Once again, I researched spinal cord terminology. The Christopher and Dana Reeve Foundation provided a wealth of information that helped me wade through issues and terms that I had never considered before. *High tone, low tone . . .* According to my previous knowledge of *tone*, it meant that someone was in good physical condition. In Hunter's case, it referred to the elasticity in his leg muscles. High tone could bring spasms and pain, and low tone could bring flaccidity. The catabolic state referred to the breakdown of muscle in Hunter's lower body. Our entire family needed to process this new information.

I sent an email after my research.

He'll get through this, and so will we. I fully expect Hunter to broaden his horizons and do more than he ever would have imagined. God has given all three of you amazing gifts of compassion and love of life that will continue to grow.

Chapter 22

Thursday, July 17

Good evening to all of you.

This has been a week of progress and turmoil for us. Hunter continues to make great strides as he works toward recovery. He can get in and out of a wheelchair with little help. He would require no help if he had use of his right hand. The broken finger and pulled tendon on that hand prevent him from putting pressure on it, which hinders him in a variety of ways.

Today, he dressed himself. I laughed when he said he missed a button and was one off all the way down. As I told him, most of us have done that with two good hands and the full use of our neck without a brace. Because he has kept in good shape and is quite nimble, he managed his pants beautifully astounding the occupational therapist.

These achievements and the very act of trying to recuperate take a great deal out of Hunter. He does not get much sleep despite the fact that he'll say he does. He turns himself every two hours at night to prevent break down of skin, so you can just imagine the toll that takes on a good night's sleep. We've been told that a cushioned foam mattress top will allow him to turn fewer times during the night, so we'll make sure to have these on the bed in Spout and in Portland.

Adapting to being a paraplegic is an overwhelming, ongoing process. It requires strength of mind, body, and spirit as well as support from many people in many ways—particularly prayers and understanding. You have to focus on yourself and your needs in order to recover. After all, who else is going to live in your body as an independent person?

The doctors took the staples out of his head yesterday and the stitches out of his back today. Both areas have healed beautifully. Hunter is looking forward to being in water again. Sponge baths are fine, but there is nothing like being in a shower to clean yourself.

Rehab is still an unknown for us. The expedited disability and Medicaid are not quite as expedited as we'd like. Like everyone else, we want things done now and government simply does not work that way. I believe once we have a place and a time, the stress level will be reduced.

I continue to stay with Hunter. While the nurses and doctors are good, this is still an institution and Hunter is particularly vulnerable right now. He has nightmares, and having me with him allows him a degree of assurance when he awakens in a strange place unable to move himself. The other night I ran to his bedside as he screamed out loud. He gave a startled shudder as he opened his eyes. I could see awareness of the disruption being a nightmare. With a groggy voice, he tried to reassure me, "It's only a nightmare. I'll be okay." As he gains more confidence in himself, his surroundings, and the people around him, this will change.

Hunter is still not up to visitors. As I mentioned before, it is very taxing trying to control the pain and be sociable. This, too, will change as the healing continues. For now, please message me if you want to drop in. I'll check with Hunter to see how he's doing and let you know if a visit will work.

Bridget and the little ones have been home this week because all three kids have colds and we don't want them to pick up anything else from the hospital, nor do we want Hunter to be exposed to anything else. Poor Bridget! It's hard having three coughing, unhappy little ones with your support group unable to help. She misses seeing Hunter, something that used to happen on a daily basis.

Boo is continuing to work with Birdie at home. He's arranging for her health care both in the health care center and once she gets back home. Michael and Evelyn are pursuing the apartment remodeling in Portland—looking into necessary permits, consulting with architect, and lining up builders.

On a lighter note, I'm a Fox News fan, especially in the evenings, and I am missing it. Hunter doesn't watch television at all and he especially doesn't like Fox News! It's a good thing I can catch news on the internet.

Thank you for your prayers. Please continue to pray for Hunter's recovery and the strength to meet the daily stressors and challenges.

"Hey, Mom, I'm tired of being in this room," Hunter told me as I finished writing. "Do you want to go for a spin around the hospital?"

"Sure." I hit Send. "That's a great idea, and I could use the exercise."

I'd pushed Hunter around the hospital before. We'd investigated areas we previously hadn't known existed in this huge edifice. Because it was a teaching hospital, there were lecture rooms and offices in addition to the countless specialty areas found in major health centers. Although I had lived in Virginia for most of my life, I had never realized how large that hospital was and how many people walked through its doors every day.

Both of us enjoyed the walls of windows that ran through much of the first floor. We could stroll through the halls and enjoy the sunshine without having to endure the overwhelming heat and humidity of a Central Virginia summer. I could only imagine how much the enclosed crosswalks meant to doctors and patients when the cold and snow of winter set in.

"Hold on a minute, Mom. Let me do a lift." Hunter interrupted my thoughts. He was determined to do his prescribed pressure-relief lifts every fifteen minutes, as his therapists had recommended. Though he could do these with the wheelchair in motion, he wasn't comfortable doing it that way. As I pulled off to the side of the hall to allow him time to exercise, I watched in admiration. He had been in such good shape before the accident, and because of that, he could lift his entire body up. I couldn't imagine too many people doing that with such ease. I couldn't.

After walking down halls and taking elevators to explore different floors and wings, I realized we'd gotten lost.

"I sure hope you know how to get back to the room," I told Hunter.

He grinned. "Hey, you're the driver. You're supposed to keep track of where we're going and how to get back."

"Then you'd better keep your eyes peeled for a nurses' station, because I don't have a clue."

Chapter 23

I continued to advocate for Hunter while preparing for the upcoming school year. The principal was concerned about my workload, which included testing new students, ordering textbooks, and formatting the master schedule into Excel. I wanted and needed to continue to do those things. They provided a sense of normalcy amid the turmoil of each day. I could manage the textbook orders and the schedule, but I could not test new students. Our middle school teacher, Susan Shorter, who was my traveling partner for our Family, Career and Community Leaders of America (FCCLA) state and national events, emailed me from Texas, where she had been with our girls for the national competition.

> *Wanted to take a minute to let you know that I'm available to help this summer in any way. Can I take a load off by ordering textbooks, or making phone calls, how about paperwork for accreditation? I plan to call Whitney, with your permission, and get her some of her textbooks, including Latin 1a. I'm willing to do what I can, my traveling is over once we land tomorrow night.*

Susan immediately became the person to administer placement tests, which took a load off my mind.

I also worked on information for one of the classes I was scheduled to teach in the fall. The leadership course was for our middle school students. Its competencies needed to be sent to the Family and Consumer Sciences specialist at the State Department of Education,

Helen Fuqua. Helen had been my sister-in-law's roommate in college. She'd seen my children when they were toddlers. We had run across each other at teachers' conferences years ago and periodically remained in contact. When I sent the competencies to Helen, she asked how my summer was going. I was sure my response was more than she expected.

I ended it with, *As I've said to many people, "Nothing and everything in my life has prepared me for this."*

Helen's response filled my heart. It reinforced my thankfulness for friends who shared in my Christian belief that prayers make a difference. I felt her love surrounding me.

Marcie,

I stopped to say a prayer for Hunter and you when I read your email this morning. I will continue to pray for Hunter and your family.

Love and prayers,

Helen

Thanks, Helen. As Hunter continues to say, "The prayers are what saved me."

With that email running through my mind, I checked our student enrollment and compared it to the chart I had for consumable textbooks and reusables we had on hand. I then began the process of ordering books, going class by class in each subject area until I had crossed off every needed text on my list. Glancing over at Hunter, I saw he had fallen asleep somewhere between the order for the penmanship books and the one for the new physics books. I closed the file and my laptop and followed his lead.

Chapter 24

Some days felt like repeats of the one before—doctors, therapists, learning new skills, and pain. As the days turned into weeks, Hunter experienced more pain and continued to have problems sleeping. I became frustrated with what I perceived as lack of progress with Medicaid, disability, and rehab. I felt for the person responsible for making sure everyone who needed help with the paperwork got it, but like anyone, I still wanted the process to be fast. Our son's health depended on it. My notes home reflected my frustration and Hunter's ongoing concern about medication.

July 18, 2014

Hunter began having pain in legs this morning. His doctor mentioned a couple of different meds for it, but Hunter said he would prefer to keep it simple with just one. The Dr. also said the physical therapy should help with the muscle pains. Hunter talked about stem cell research and the doctors seem to think it's a lot closer than we thought.

Still waiting to talk with the caseworker—she's been gone every time I poke my head out to find her.

I finally heard from the Appomattox Social Services person in charge of Medicaid. Appomattox has not received the disability approval, which means that they can't process the Medicaid. UVA is responsible for facilitating the disability and that hasn't happened.

So I'm trying to touch base with the caseworker to start pushing from this end. It looks like next week will be the earliest we find out about rehab . . .

Hunter still gets little sleep. Eventually, he's going to have to crash. He's still absorbing so much that it is difficult to sleep.

July 21

Good afternoon.

I hope all of you had a great weekend and a good start to a new week.

Hunter continues to progress but also to have a lot of pain—in his entire body. The doctor suggested a different medicine that Aunt Carol M. checked out for Hunter. She found that he could take it with little worry. He's holding off until he absolutely feels he needs it.

Hunter had both physical and occupational therapy today. I suppose I should say I also had occupational therapy today.

I had to change Hunter's neck brace. I was terrified. It had to be taken off totally with him lying perfectly still. In my mind, I was crying to God, "Oh, my God. Oh, my God. Oh, my God. Help me please." Silent tears were pouring down my face as I relived holding Hunter's bleeding head on the road. I asked God to help me change the pads quickly and to replace the neck brace perfectly. It was daunting to think that one wrong move on my part could cause further damage to Hunter.

The awful thing is that I am supposed to remove the neck brace daily to check his skin for lesions. I can tell you that the hospital staff has not been doing that—probably because the nurses are just as frightened as I am.

Nothing and everything in my life has prepared me for this and all the challenges of the past two weeks.

On the good news side, I spoke with two social workers this afternoon. One checked on the disability aspect and found out that it is currently with social security. The expectation is that it should be determined by tomorrow and will be sent to Medicaid. The other social worker does rehab and said the message she received this morning is that Hunter will be accepted into HealthSouth. Her caveat was that it might change. I am greatly encouraged because this is the first that HealthSouth says they will take him. I can only think that is because a couple of the docs here work with HealthSouth and have put in the word that Hunter is an outstanding patient with a great attitude, hence an excellent candidate for them. My prayer is that all of this will work out quickly. I try to remain faithful. More good news is that the rehab doc said that a lot of the pain in Hunter's back is due to him working so hard that the muscles are knotting. She gave him a massage, which helped immensely. He also has heating pads to help with the muscle pain. And he can sleep on his belly, which is his preferred way of sleeping. I'm hoping that will allow him a more natural sleep that is a bit longer in length.

The work of learning how to use a wheelchair, how to dress without use of your lower body, and how to hold your neck perfectly still so your mom can change your neck brace correctly is exhausting. While Hunter feels like he could visit with family members for short periods of time, he does not feel up to visiting with others yet. If you're an aunt, uncle, cousin, grandma and have some time and would like to stop in, text me, email me, or call so I can tell you how the day is looking. Just don't invite any friends to come with you. It is difficult enough adapting to being a paraplegic without having people you don't know well in your room.

Thank you for your continuing prayers and support. We all continue to need them

With love,

Marcie

As with many of my other emails, this one brought several responses. Some provided insight into the nature of pain and healing; others included words of encouragement.

Hey Marcie and Hunter,

Wish I could have been there to help with the neck brace change. They should have been doing it all along. Hunter doesn't need any added healing to deal with.

It is important for Hunter to take his pain or anti-inflammatory meds as prescribed to maintain a constant level of med. That will keep his pain level at a low enough level to help him heal. Waiting until he is in pain to take a med is stressful for his body. The focus should be on rest & healing, which the meds can help with.

This is just my 2 cents worth from a loving & concerned Aunt Janet. Our love and prayers continue to be with all of you. Onward & upward.

OMG, Marcie, I would be feeling the same way about putting on his neck brace!!!! Hunter called me on Saturday and we talked for about 45 mins. He sounds upbeat and practical at the same time. You/Hunter/all have been on a surreal journey over the last two weeks.

I will be in Richmond on the night of July 31 and will stay until August 10, so I hope to get up and visit you/Hunter/Bridget . . . we'll see what Hunter will be up for in a few weeks.

Love you, Marcie, and thank you for keeping us all so well informed!

Xoxox,

Sally

I know you are terrified but what a good job you are doing. Please remember that the human body is more resilient than we think. Each time you change a bandage it will get easier and easier. I am still planning to be in Charlottesville this weekend. I will keep posted as to where to go. I love you and can't wait to see you and Hunter and family.

    Janis

During one of the quieter times of our day, I found myself watching my cherished son as he slept through his pain. I wondered about his future—our future. The paranoia and mania that I had caught glimpses of early in his hospitalization seemed to have disappeared. I was so grateful for that, but I also feared that it could return. I firmly believed that I would recognize early symptoms and would not hesitate to seek help, but for now I wanted to tamp down my fear. I reminded myself that worrying was not going to change a thing. Once again, I needed to trust the Lord.

Chapter 25

My mother was not much of an emailer, but she called several times during the first few weeks of Hunter's stay at the hospital. During one of those phone calls, we recalled her always encouraging my siblings and me to put our faith in God, and how my faith in him had helped me to accept the challenges of the past weeks.

"I don't know how anyone can make it through these situations without help from God," I told her. "I know a lot of people have a hard time believing that a loving God would allow bad things to happen, and I have read several articles about this, but I have come to the same conclusion every time—I am one of those people who doesn't need to know why these things happen. I need the courage and faith to make my way through them."

It turned out that she already knew this about me.

"Marcie," she said, "it is your faith in God's plans that will always help you get through any situation."

Shortly after this conversation with my mother, my Aunt Kathryn sent me an email on the same topic.

Dear Marcie,

God gives special blessings to people who are called upon to do things in their lives that they never anticipated. You and Hunter will come through this period and one day will look back on these days and wonder how you ever made it through. We all have within us the ability to respond to whatever happens in our lives; we learn to cope . . . We all have strengths within us that we are not aware of until some event pulls us up short and we somehow manage to cope and do whatever it takes at the time. From your emails I can ascertain that you are doing beautifully. With God's help and the love and caring wishes from all your friend and family, this too shall pass. Tell Hunter he has more friends and family wanting him well and to be among us than he can possibly imagine. Keep up the good work!

Love, Aunt Kathryn

Aunt Kathryn's message touched my heart. It reminded me that difficult experiences oftentimes enable us to help others, both in the future and in the midst of our pain. Her email brought to mind a recent encounter I'd had.

I had told Hunter that I thought he was doing well enough for me to walk down the hall to the family room to watch a television program, and I left him talking on the phone to my sister Janis. When I got to the room, I saw a woman sitting in a chair, obviously distraught, so I started talking with her.

Simone was from Georgia and had been in Virginia for two weeks. Her twenty-three-year-old daughter ended up in the hospital in Reston because of vocal cord paralysis and lung problems. After two weeks filled with numerous tests but no answers, the doctors decided to move her to UVA. Her mom followed the ambulance, driving on fumes and prayers.

Simone told me about her belief in God and admitted that she wondered how all this could be happening. Her friends offered platitudes but didn't understand the depth of her anguish. Having spent the past two-plus weeks watching our son struggle, I understood Simone's struggle to the bottom of my soul. I listened, talked with her, held her hand while she cried, soothed her fears, and prayed for her and her daughter. I didn't get to watch the program, but I had the opportunity to reaffirm to this believing mother that God was indeed with her.

As I walked back to Hunter's room, I sent up a quick prayer. *Thank you, Lord, for allowing me to spend time with Simone. You knew it would fill my soul to be able to help another mother.*

Chapter 26

Despite our closeness, my family began to crack under the strain of our long ordeal. In addition to concerns about Hunter's recovery, we wondered where he was going to live, how he would cope, and how to move forward as a family. The delays in getting answers to our many questions wore on us. I had done everything I could do. It was a matter of waiting, which had never been one of my strengths.

"You just need to stay on them, Marcie," my husband said impatiently during one of our numerous calls about the lack of progress.

"I have been!" I snapped back. I felt my good mood evaporating with the stress of little sleep and lots of worry. While disagreeing about things might have been normal for couples, I still didn't like it. I just wanted to know what to expect.

Even if the Portland move worked out, Hunter still needed a place to stay after rehab. He would not be able to go to Portland for several months, as it would take at least that long to make the changes to Michael's house. Hunter couldn't go back to his old house, as it was not handicap accessible. The only possible place for him to move was back home. He wanted and needed to be more independent, but he also recognized that he would need help for quite some time.

We considered and discarded various plans for our house. Boo suggested enclosing part of our front porch to make a bedroom for Hunter, but that would block the entrance to our house. We considered making our large walk-in closet into a bedroom, but Hunter wouldn't have privacy. I finally thought of a solution that I hoped would work for all of us and presented it in an email to Boo, Michael, and Bridget.

I do want Michael and Bridget to be aware of my thinking and why I am requesting this consideration. I am not including Hunter because he has so much on his plate right now that he does not need one more thing.

I have been thinking and praying about the changes that will naturally occur when Hunter comes to stay with us. I know that we decided he should use our room, and if that is what happens, then that is what happens. However, I really think we should consider closing in the small portion of the porch and moving the washer and dryer and putting in a shower unit.

There are several reasons for this continuing to be on my mind, all of which have to do with seeing the requirements that will be needed for Hunter even after rehab. Ours is the practice house—the place where he learns how to manage more independently. But he is going to need help. He is not going to come out of rehab able to do everything by himself and for himself.

First (and selfishly)—I think you and I will be more comfortable and have less stress by being in our own room. There is going to be a lot of change for us, even if for only two or three months. Keep in mind that three months is a quarter of a year. That is a long time.

Second—we are going to have to totally change our room if Hunter stays there—from the bed to the things he will need with the bed to the dressers to the office items—all of these will have to be moved. The room will by necessity have to be only Hunter's for the time he is with us. We will not be able to waltz in at will. He will need to have respect shown as he tries to take in all the new ways of taking care of himself. Even the bathroom will require changes. The door to the shower will most likely have to be removed because it will not hold Hunter as he tries to get into the shower. A curtain will have to be put up to keep water in. We'll probably need an additional shower seat. Toilet will need to have handles, so he can get on and off with relative ease.

Third—I think everyone will be better able to adapt in the fall if Hunter is in his own section of the house and can have a degree of freedom by simply wheeling himself out the door without disturbing us.

Fourth—It will make things easier for him to have some of his friends visit if they can walk into a place that is his. He will need some friends this fall, and by having a section of the house to himself, he will feel freer to socialize. I can already tell you that he is embarrassed to have folks other than family see him. The time he spends with us will help him to adjust on a level that will enable him to greet the world with enthusiasm.

Fifth—The room will always be there for Hunter for future visits. We may not be thinking about these visits now, but if he has his own room when he comes, the visits will be more normal rather than using our room. And it is very likely that Michael and Evelyn will come for some of these same visits—think Christmas—so they will need the large room upstairs, especially if we have Christmases like this past one with even more family.

Sixth—It would be nice to have a small TV room/office on the first floor. Knee surgery is a very real prospect for me in the next couple of years. We both know that I have a difficult time with steps and have had for the past few years. Your knees are also showing signs of deterioration, so a first-floor room would benefit you also.

I understand very clearly that cost is an issue. In both the short term and the long term, the cost of the room will be dwarfed by the benefits of it.

I think this could be done in the next five to six weeks since it is a room and not an entire apartment.

So please, consider this and let me know.

Michael liked the idea but was concerned about the cost and the time needed for making the necessary changes. Bridget, while also aware of the cost, had additional thoughts about the suggestion. She quickly emailed her response.

Great reasons. I think it is very important for Mama and Daddy to "have a place" that Hunter can call home. If even for a few months, and then a few weeks out of the years he'll always know he can come and visit easily without kicking anybody out of their room. I think it's important for him to feel welcome and not to feel like he's being a burden to anybody.

I'm not a contractor nor have I had much to do with additions/ renovations, but when I think about it, I really don't see it costing much more than $5k. I think that at least getting an estimate is a good idea so it's not just a guessing game with numbers.

Just my 2 cents. Much cheaper than paying for a funeral, which I fully believe almost happened. Hunter is our miracle.

My husband replied that he had contacted two contractors. Knowing that he had taken action so quickly brought some relief to the ever-present gnawing in my stomach.

Chapter 27

I found a rare quiet moment in the afternoon to tell Hunter about the family's plan. "I sent your dad an email about an idea I had for making a room for you at the house."

"What's your idea?" he asked.

"I want to take the hot tub out and move the laundry room there. Then I want to enclose the back porch area behind the current laundry room and turn it into a bedroom for you. We can add a shower to the half-bath to give you your own small suite."

Hunter was pleased with these new suggestions and sent an email to his dad.

> *I'll be able to give u more info by Mon. We just got approval for HealthSouth.*
>
> *Noon tomorrow is my xfer time.*
>
> *Sounds like a wonderful place. I'm excited.*
>
> *I'm hoping bigger is better, but I'm a minimalistic person. Mom just informed me of your remodel plans, I am grateful. Thank you.*
>
> *Know that my paralysis is but a temporary event, someday in the future, whether it's ten, twenty or more years, this too shall pass.*
>
> *Love, Hunter*

Tears welled up as I read the note. The accident had not changed his positive, uplifting spirit. He was the Hunter I remembered. He absolutely believed that, at some point, science would find a cure for paraplegics. He had already read online articles about advances in spinal cord injuries and relayed the information not only to me as we passed time in the hospital room, but also to his doctors. He wanted to gain as much knowledge as possible about what was going on in the field, and he wanted to hear the opinions of the experts assigned to his case.

"Hey, Mom," he said, glancing up from his computer. "Check out this article. I'll send you the link."

"Okay," I replied. "What's this one about?"

"It's about some experiments researchers are doing with stimulating the nerves in the spinal cord. They're doing some medical trials. I wish I met the criteria. I'd volunteer."

"That would be amazing." I wished there was a way to get him in a trial study. Maybe someday.

Hunter religiously asked his doctors about the meds they prescribed, the therapy they recommended, and the long-term possibilities for someone like him—a T12 complete. As I listened to the conversations, I realized that many patients probably didn't pose questions like Hunter's. He had a thirst for knowledge and an intellect to match that thirst.

With the move to rehab on the horizon, we considered power of attorney. After discussing this with Hunter, we gathered information about it and exchanged numerous emails in the process. The requirements in Virginia versus Oregon became the focus as we determined what to do for both the short and long term.

After talking with some lawyer friends, we discovered that the Commonwealth of Virginia had a form called the Virginia Advance Medical Directive. According to the directive, "You have the right to name someone to make health care decisions for you if you are unable to make them of yourself. You have the right to give instructions about what types of health care you want or do not want. You may use this whole form or any part to tell your wishes." These were sobering words. It hurt to think that one of my children needed to complete this.

Hunter's handwriting still wasn't up to par, so I completed the basic information on the form, and Hunter read it, crossed out, and initialed the parts he did not want to relinquish to the POA, and signed it. Two of the hospital personnel witnessed his signature and signed as well. With little fanfare, I became the primary agent and Bridget became the substitute agent. A heavy cloak of responsibility enshrouded me. *Please, Lord, continue to heal Hunter so he can take care of himself. And I ask that you continue to guide Bridget and me as we serve as his advocates through this process. Thank you for always being with us.*

Chapter 28

On July 25, life changed again.

We had great news about Hunter today—for about 30 minutes.

All the paperwork came through and he had been accepted into UVA's HealthSouth Rehab. He was scheduled for transport at noon tomorrow. We were all so excited to be able to take this next step.

However, the bubble burst when the results of the latest spinal x-ray came in. The x-ray showed that something was different about the spine, so a CT scan was ordered. The scan confirmed that there was a loose screw in the L3 and that there was a compression fracture in the L4. So . . . another surgery is being scheduled to repair both.

Not sure when the surgery will take place—hopefully at the beginning of the week.

Hunter is now confined to a 30-degree elevation in bed until further notice. No wheelchair, no physical therapy, nothing that may cause further injury to the L4.

His spirit is amazing. He simply says that it's better this was discovered before he got to rehab so that it can be repaired quickly and efficiently. I must say I agree—I can't imagine him getting to rehab only to have this kind of setback.

The Lord continues to take care of Hunter. Please keep him in your prayers as he goes through another surgery and recovery period.

My spirits plummeted at the unexpected news of another surgery. Hunter had been making such great strides. He could get himself out of bed and into the wheelchair, dress himself, insert his own catheter, and so much more. The x-ray had been standard procedure for patients before going to rehab—one more item to check off the list before making the move. We'd started the day elated to be going to HealthSouth. It had a good reputation and was close to Hunter's doctors in Charlottesville, only ninety minutes from home. And now this.

One of the nurses told me that the loose screw caused the compression fracture. But what caused the screw to loosen in a paraplegic with limited mobility? Regardless of the cause, the consequence was the same—another surgery.

July 26,

Surgery is scheduled for tomorrow. Not certain of the time.

It turns out this is another major surgery. They'll replace the original rods and screws and add more in the L area. They also plan to put metal plates in his hips to strengthen them. Please pray that the surgery goes well, that there are no further complications, and that recovery is smooth and quick.

Hunter continues to be positive and grateful that the compression fracture was found now rather than later.

Boo, Michael, Bridget, and I texted throughout the day of Hunter's back surgery.

Just talked to unit nurse and then surgery nurse—surgery began at 9:36. Will last 4–6 hours. He'll go to NEURO ICU for a day or two then come back to 6WEST. So far, everything is going well. No blood has been needed. I'm packing up my things for the car and then his things, as we have to vacate this room since he will be in ICU. We can't stay in ICU, so I plan to be home later tonight.

Michael asked that I continue to update them on the surgery as I acquired new information, and Bridget wanted to make certain that I could stay until Hunter was out of surgery.

Sure, I'll stay until I'm sure he's okay. They're not pushing me out of room. I'm trying to stay ahead of request to vacate

Her reply came quickly: *Ok, good :).*
She wrote again. *He knows you can't stay night in ICU, right?*
I told her . . .*Not sure if he knows that.*

Reading while Hunter underwent this surgery proved to be impossible. After perusing the same paragraph five times, I gave up and put the book away. Once again, I took to walking the hospital grounds for stress relief.

Finally, I was able to send my family an update.

He's out of surgery. Everything went well. Only took out screws on L4—everything above looked really good. Put screws in L5, S1, and iliac bone (pelvic, hip). He's awake, talking, and ready for me to come back. He's in 6th floor Neuro ICU.

Michael wrote back first. *Hooray! So glad to hear things went well! Now for another round of healing! Thanks for being there mom!*
I replied immediately. *I'm glad to be able to be here.*
Bridget joined the conversation. *Amen.*
With that final *Amen* of Bridget's echoing in my head, I began my walk to Hunter's new room.

Chapter 29

Once the sedation wore off, Hunter sent out his own email. He had been Snapchatting with siblings, cousins, and friends before the surgery and picked up exactly where he left off.

All titanium was added, I'm in ICU the next day or 2 on the 6th floor, then back to 6 west.

I'm allowed h2o now, dark liquids later, then food etc.

Pain wise, not bad, burning pain on incision skin, I'm rotating side to side every 2 hours, to maximize o2 to wound

10 mg oxy, every 3 hours.

Mom's here, she will stay til 7 pm or so when hospital sitter comes in, Mom will be back in the morning.

Prayer/positive intention wise, please focus on peace and health for all.

Visitor wise if you are on this email list, you have an open invite, all blood and marriage folks have an open invite; however, do not bring anyone else with you, thank you.

Know that I am in no need of visitors; this is purely to satisfy your desires ;)

I will let you know more as it develops, if you want off this list let me know

I will email more updates as they develop.

Thanks,

Hunter

I shook my head in amusement when I read, *Know that I am in no need of visitors, this is purely to satisfy your desires.* That was pure Hunter. He had not felt up to visitors the first few weeks, but after learning how many people asked about visiting and how important it seemed to them, he realized that they needed to see him—that it would make them feel better. While he healed physically and emotionally, he understood that seeing him helped family and close friends to also heal.

The hospital routine of daily doctor visits and physical and occupational therapy resumed quickly. This time, we knew what to expect. Our goal was to move to rehab as soon as possible. We felt ready for the next phase of recovery and could not hide our eagerness.

"Bridget, I don't know how people endure hospital stays that last for months," I told my daughter when I walked her and the children back to the van after a visit with Hunter. "We've been here over three and a half weeks, and I cannot wait to leave. Hunter is literally chomping at the bit to move to rehab."

"I know," she replied. "It feels like months, not just weeks."

"Exactly!" I loved having a daughter who knew how I felt. Her empathy was exactly what I needed at that moment.

The medical personnel had been wonderful, but Hunter and I had hit the point where we needed to move on. Knowing that rehab was just around the corner only increased our desire to fast-forward the days.

Hunter's doctor ordered one more MRI to verify that the screws were tight before giving the green light for moving to rehab. I wanted to do a happy dance when the results came back. We were on the way to HealthSouth! I packed up the items I'd brought from home and Hunter's things and waited impatiently for the ambulance service to arrive. The plan was for me to meet him at HealthSouth and stay a few days while he adjusted to a new facility. He was still having nightmares and had become accustomed to having me with him. This would eventually change, but for now I was like a security blanket. He counted on me to bring him the organic food he would eat—one thing that hospitals did not cater to. His nutritional needs had changed with the paralysis, limiting his total fluid intake, so we needed to make certain that everything he ate was nutrient packed. His determination to follow all of the doctor's instructions amazed me.

"You're here!" Hunter said in relief when the ambulance service arrived in his room to transfer him to HealthSouth. "Let's get me out of here. They've been great, but I am ready to leave."

The crew gently moved Hunter from bed to gurney as he reminded them to be careful because he didn't want any of the pins in his back jostled—which would require another surgery.

He looked up at me. "I'll see you in a while, Mom."

"Yes, you will!" I replied in a choked voice. My heart ached as I held in tears of joy. *Thank you, Lord, for bringing us this far. Please continue to guard my son.*

Chapter 30

Y*our road to recovery starts here.* The logo embossed on the floor of HealthSouth hit me smack in the face with its veracity. My eyes overflowed. It had been a long twenty-seven days, and we'd made it this far. The Lord answered my prayer for strength to handle whatever came my way. Now the next step in the journey was beginning.

Hunter had a private room with two beds. I would actually be able to sleep in a real bed! While I was grateful to be allowed to stay with Hunter at the hospital, I felt even more grateful to have that bed.

We met his nurses and therapists. I could see his anxiety level rising again. That didn't surprise me, given all he'd been through, but knowing I could only stay long enough to get him settled made us nervous. We had grown accustomed to me helping Hunter in the numerous things that required an extra hand, from the small tasks like retrieving a fallen pencil to getting his food from the refrigerator. It eased the stress of his daily living. He would now learn to handle those things himself as he faced the courageous step of starting anew.

Friday, August 1

> *Subject: Update from Hunter's Mama*
>
> *HOORAY! We're at UVA's HealthSouth!*
>
> *Hunter has spent the days since his Sunday surgery in ICU, Neuro Step Down, and Acute Care at UVA. He was transported*

to HealthSouth late this afternoon and feels like he's in a luxury hotel. He's already scheduled to begin his rehab program tomorrow. He'll spend three hours in actual training on Saturday and Sunday. Monday, he'll bump up to six hours a day! Quite a workout.

Please continue to keep him in prayer as he continues his journey to recovery. He's still in quite a bit of pain but manages it better than most people. Of course, he still has the staples in his back from the latest surgery.

His positive attitude and sense of humor preceded his physical presence in HealthSouth. The doctors and nurses have all told him that they have heard so many good things about him and are so glad to have him here with them. His primary doctor finished his checkup by telling him that he was happy to serve Hunter. Reminded me of our wonderful CCA staff.

Hunter's new room was huge compared to the one at the hospital. He had a view of an appealing grassy commons. His new nurse was warm and inviting and gave us a tour of the floor, which included a lounge area with a kitchenette-style nook and a rehab room filled with machines and tools designed to help people with various physical challenges. Hunter's face lit up at the sight of so much equipment. He was ready to take on the world. I breathed a sigh of satisfaction as we settled into this new facility.

Boo, Bridget, and the children made their almost daily trek to HealthSouth to see Hunter and his new temporary abode. Etta and Hans loved seeing him and his room. He showed everyone the small kitchen area on his floor and the rehab room. The facility had a sitting area with a television and newspapers. The elevators allowed Hunter to take the children outside and all of us to take short walks around the building.

The days I spent with Hunter at HealthSouth were filled with activity. His daily regimen included physical and occupational sessions that would help him adjust to life outside of an institution. The nurse made it clear that I did not need to be around for these.

"Good luck with your sessions, Hunter," I said as I headed to the elevator.

"Be careful driving, Mom," he told me. "I'll see you tonight."

With those words, I headed home to do the ordinary things in life that had been relegated to lesser importance over the past month. I cooked. I cleaned. I puttered. I savored every minute of these mundane tasks. Then I headed back to spend the night with my son.

Hunter developed a strong rapport with his new doctor and looked forward to seeing him and peppering him with questions.

"What do you think about electric stimulation for paralysis?"

And off they would go, discussing the latest research in spinal cord injuries.

He enjoyed his new therapists and found that they helped him in unexpected ways. Using their equipment and training, they focused on what needed to be done to promote the overall physical and emotional health of their patients. While he still experienced manic symptoms such as talking nonstop, Hunter's mental health seemed stable.

I had a harder time transitioning back home than Hunter did seeing me go. Despite the fact that I knew he was in good hands, I felt like I should be with him. I also understood that Hunter needed to be on his own, not have him mom with him on a daily basis.

Saturday, August 16

Subject: Update from Hunter's Mama

It's been two weeks since Hunter entered rehab at UVA's HealthSouth. He has made so much progress that even the doctors and nurses are impressed.

I stayed the first four nights at rehab with him. After that, I drove up daily. Now, I'm on the every-other-day visitation schedule. I am grateful to be a school administrator who can do so much of the job via computer. Our teaching staff begins Monday and I will be back at school full time.

Hunter's back stitches are gone (steri strips are still in place). He is healing beautifully.

His hand brace was removed Thursday. He now has a brace for his finger and is able to use his hand to help maneuver. The pins in the hand can be removed whenever Hunter chooses.

It will take around four months for the bone to fuse itself to the rods and pins, so Hunter has to be very careful with his movements. No bending, lifting, or twisting.

He's doing a wonderful job of transferring himself from the bed to the wheelchair. It's amazing to see how proficient he has become at this in just two short weeks.

Yesterday, Bridget, the children and I went to see Hunter. I dropped off Bridget, so she and Hunter could have some brother-sister time (and Sebastian time) while I took Etta and Hans to Whole Foods to get some organic whole milk yogurt for Hunter. When the little ones and I walked into the building, Bridget was strolling Sebastian down the hall and Hunter was wheeling himself—hand gloves and all. Etta and Hans ran to their uncle calling his name. As we walked the grounds, Etta said, "Uncle Hunter can do anything now." Seeing their uncle pushing himself around with such vitality was the greatest gift for our two little ones.

On the home front, we are working hard to prepare the room and bathroom for Hunter's return home, which could be within two weeks. We have had some great help from different people—Dave Doss, Chris Jones, Dave and D. C. Matthews, Marcus Neale, Bridget Jones Neale, Geoff Hubler, and the Liberty Baptist Church Compassion Ministry Team. The Liberty men built the most wonderful ramp for Hunter in a little over a day. Amazing. We are so grateful to these folks who are helping us. (I'm attaching a pic of some of the Liberty team with our grandson on the ramp.)

I thank you for your prayers and ask that you continue to remember us in your daily talks with the Lord. The prayers have helped us as we have met the daily challenges in our lives. God is good.

Chapter 31

Wednesday, August 27, marked another big day for us. We took Hunter home from rehab.

"Uncle Hunter, Uncle Hunter," Etta and Hans yelled and ran up to him as soon as we got him out of the vehicle.

Hunter reached out to give them a squeeze. He could never pick them up again, but he could hold their small hands in his large ones.

"See your new ramp?" Hans pointed to it. "The men came and built it for you."

"Look at your new room," called out Etta. "You can't sleep in there yet because the door's not fixed. Papa says it won't be long before it's ready for you. You get to have a sleepover in the living room until then."

"I see," Hunter replied as he took in his niece's and nephew's excitement. "Maybe you can help your mama and Gaga put my things away for me."

And off they went, eager to help their uncle.

Each day out of the hospital felt like a gift to all of us. Every hour brought something new. Hunter was pretty independent but still needed someone to help with things like laundry and fetching out-of-reach items. Simple things we took for granted and did quickly required a great deal of effort from him. His positive attitude and desire to be totally independent served him well.

Bridget and the children visited often, which helped him maintain his upbeat outlook. Hans was fascinated with some of Hunter's tools, such as the grabber. He loved to use it whenever he was at the house. He and Etta occasionally squabbled over whose turn it was to try it out.

"Mama, Hans won't share Uncle Hunter's grabber," Etta complained to Bridget.

"It's not a toy," Bridget reminded her. "You both need to be careful with that. Uncle Hunter needs it to pick up things."

"I'm going to order one for each of them," Hunter quickly decided. "I think I can find cheap ones online."

The wheels on Hunter's chair captivated Sebastian. He sat in his walker and reached out to touch them whenever Hunter sat next to him. He even started chasing Hunter around the room. Watching a ten-month-old in his walker running after his uncle in his wheelchair provided welcome laughter.

After Hunter was home a few days, Etta asked him to come visit her classroom at school. "If you want to," she told him in earnestness.

Hunter had been in her school before, just not in a wheelchair. In Etta's eyes, the wheelchair did not change a thing about her uncle. She did not view it as a barrier. It was simply the way he moved from place to place.

Once again I was reminded that the Lord uses even the smallest in his kingdom to open the eyes and hearts of his people.

Thank you, Lord.

Epilogue

The four and a half years since Hunter's accident have been filled with the stresses and joys of living. Tempers have flared, and laughter has filled our home. Hunter's journey to recovery continues to this day. He believes that there will be a cure for paralysis, so he takes care of himself in the hope that he will eventually benefit from it.

The first few months he was home, I found myself waking in the middle of the night, praying for Hunter. *Please, God, be with Hunter*, I pleaded. *Bless him and keep him, make your face to shine upon him and be gracious to him, lift up your countenance on him and give him peace.* This personalization of Numbers 6 reflected my feelings so accurately, and it brought me the peace that I wished for Hunter. While I no longer awaken during the night, I continue to keep Hunter and all my family in prayer.

Bridget became Hunter's primary source of help. He no longer wanted my aid; he needed and wanted help from his sister. They had always had a close relationship, but the accident deepened it. Instead of Hunter walking to her house and playing with the children, Bridget came to our house and helped him with everyday tasks, such as changing sheets and sweeping and simply listening to him as only a sibling can. The move to Portland didn't work out as we'd hoped. After months of lamenting the fact that he wanted to move and to be independent, Hunter pulled on his reservoir of determination and faith and made the decision to travel while his health still allowed it. His mentor and former teacher, Barry Sauls, had told him that he was the only one holding himself back from taking that first step, so he went for it.

Hunter has visited states from Virginia to California, camping out in his hand-controlled van and enjoying the beauty of God's world. He sent texts home to let us know where he was and how he was, and he called when he had good phone reception. He came home for Christmas and is making plans for his next excursion.

While I no longer feel like I am shattering, I still relive Hunter's accident. It only takes a screech of brakes on a television show or a thud when one object connects with another to throw my mind back in time. Like me, Bridget also relives that July 4. My husband handles it in his quiet way, while Michael copes with the guilt he feels over having so many blessings while his brother lives in pain.

Over time Hunter has lost some memories of the accident. He has gaps in his memory from before and after that day. So far he has not shown any sign of another psychotic break, and I can guarantee that we've stayed alert to any red flags. In the course of several talks with Hunter about the break and his mental health, he has posed the question, "Could the total severance of the spinal cord and the head trauma have caused the chemical imbalance to somehow change?"

I have no answer for that.

My hope and my prayer is that the Lord allows me the opportunity to use my experiences to help someone else as she finds herself in the midst of crisis. May he let my pain ease someone else's so I can comfort another as the Lord comforted me during those dark days of summer when I thought I might shatter.

Praise to the God of all comfort. "Praise be to the God and Father of our Lord Jesus Christ, the Father of compassion and the God of all comfort, who comforts us in all our troubles, so that we can comfort those in any trouble with the comfort we ourselves receive from God" (2 Corinthians 1:3–4 NIV).

Acknowledgments

S*hattering* is a story, a family story, a personal story I wanted to share. It was not easy to write, but it was necessary. Mental illness is not a choice we make, but rather a challenge we face. We all handle it differently. A spinal cord injury is also not a choice we make. It is a challenge we face. Like mental illness, we all handle it differently. Our family has been blessed in so many ways through our experiences.

I am grateful for my husband's love and support in making *Shattering* a reality. Without Boo, it would not be. I am also grateful for the support of my children and their spouses—Michael and Evelyn, Bridget and Marcus, and Hunter. You accepted my desire to share our story without hesitation. I am particularly grateful to you, Bridget. You allowed me to pick your brain as I ran into questions, and you read drafts without complaint. Your confidence in me is humbling. To my wonderful grandchildren, Etta, Hans, Sebastian, and Della—your unconditional love and acceptance of your uncle Hunter melts my heart. God has blessed me with having you in my life.

My parents, John and Fran Shinholser, have been with us since the first phone call from Hawaii. My brothers and sisters and their spouses have also provided unwavering support. So here's to all of you—David and Janet Shinholser, Sally Valentine, Janis Kouche, Steven and Keller Shinholser, John and Carol Shinholser, Peter Shinholser, and Joe and Kathy Burgess. Mama, Sally, Janis, and Kathy—thank you for your many readings of the manuscript in all its stages of development. Having your constant encouragement has been a blessing.

Birdie Harvey and Mary Lou Harvey, thank you for your ongoing support.

I appreciate the help of the many doctors and nurses we have met through the years. These men and women helped Hunter as he sought recovery from mental illness and spinal cord injury. Their dedication to all of their patients is amazing.

I am grateful for the expertise of the folks at Redemption Press. Thank you to Jeanette Hanscome and Dori Harrell for the suggestions you offered that made my writing better. Thanks to Colleen Jones for keeping everything on track. And thank you to Athena Dean Holtz for providing me with the opportunity to share *Shattering*.

I tried to be as accurate as possible in writing our story. I hope that it touches other families in similar circumstances and lets them know they are not alone in their journeys. God's grace helped me each and every day. I give Him the glory.

I end with Hunter—you are loved beyond measure.

Online Resources

Through the years, I have tried to learn as much as possible about mental illness and spinal cord injuries. I am including several websites that may be helpful to those taking on their own searches.

Spinal Cord Injury Websites:

Christopher & Dana Reeve Foundation
https://www.christopherreeve.org

United Spinal Association
https://www.unitedspinal.org

SCI-INFO-PAGES
https://www.sci-info-pages.com

Paralyzed Veterans of America
https://www.pva.org

Mental Illness Websites:

NAMI
National Alliance on Mental Illness
https://www.nami.org/

Focus on the Family
https://www.focusonthefamily.com/lifechallenges/promos/mental-health-resources

National Institute of Mental Health
https://www.nimh.nih.gov/index.shtml

Mental Health America
https://www.mentalhealthamerica.net

Order Information

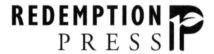

To order additional copies of this book, please visit
www.redemption-press.com.
Also available on Amazon.com and BarnesandNoble.com
Or by calling toll free 1-844-2REDEEM.

CPSIA information can be obtained
at www.ICGtesting.com
Printed in the USA
FSHW011517160419